Clinical Effectiveness and Primary Care

Mark Baker
Medical Director, North Yorkshire Health Authority and
External Professor of Public Health, University of Leeds

Neal Maskrey
Consultant in Primary Care Development, North Yorkshire
Health Authority

and

Simon Kirk
Development Manager, North Yorkshire Health Authority

Foreword by
Professor Allen Hutchinson
Chair, RCGP Quality Improvement Group

RADCLIFFE MEDICAL PRESS

© 1997 Mark Baker, Neal Maskrey and Simon Kirk

Radcliffe Medical Press Ltd
18 Marcham Road, Abingdon, Oxon OX14 1AA, UK

Radcliffe Medical Press, Inc.
141 Fifth Avenue, New York, NY 10010, USA

British Library Cataloguing in Publication Data

A catalogue record for this book is available from the British Library.

ISBN 1 85775 129 9

Library of Congress Cataloging-in-Publication Data is available.

Typeset by Advance Typesetting Ltd, Oxfordshire
Printed and bound by Biddles Ltd, Guildford and King's Lynn

Contents

About the authors

Professor Mark Baker Mark Baker is the Medical Director of North Yorkshire Health Authority, External Professor of Public Health in the School of Medicine at Leeds University and Honorary Professor of Public Health at the University of Bradford. A former trust Chief Executive and Regional Director of Research and Development, he has 16 years' experience in senior NHS management and has written extensively on health issues. He is co-editor, with Simon Kirk, of *Research and Development for the NHS*.[1]

Dr Neal Maskrey After GP vocational training in Hull, Neal Maskrey was a general practitioner and vocational training course organizer in Scarborough. In 1993 he became Medical Director of North Yorkshire Family Health Services Authority and is now Consultant in Primary Care Development for North Yorkshire Health Authority. He is also a GP assistant in Bridlington, East Yorkshire, continues to have a keen interest in GP postgraduate education, organizes regional MRCGP preparation courses and is the author of *The MRCGP Workbook*.[2]

Simon Kirk Simon Kirk joined the NHS as a research assistant at the National Association of Health Authorities. He moved to the Yorkshire Regional Health Authority, working in health promotion and public health, later becoming Regional Research and Development Information Manager. He is currently a Development Manager with North Yorkshire Health Authority.

References

1 Baker M and Kirk S (1996) *Research and Development for the NHS*. Radcliffe Medical Press, Oxford.
2 Maskrey N (1994) *The MRCGP Workbook*. Churchill Livingstone, London.

Foreword

When health policy analysts of the 21st century look back over the first 50 years of the NHS they will see four extraordinary features. First, of course, is the institution of the NHS itself, with its comprehensive services free at the point of entry. Second will be the inexorable demand for more services and ever newer and better technology, against a background of above inflation growth in resources which have failed to satisfy the population's need for care. Improved health and increasing longevity will be the third feature, in which the NHS has played a distinguished part, assisted by the effects of a general – though by no means universal – rise in affluence and quality of life.

But it is specifically to the 1990s that analysts will look to see the remarkable changes that have come about in the influence of primary care, on what has, for most of the first 50 years, been a hospital dominated system. As never before, primary care professionals – and general practitioners particularly – find themselves jumping into (or being pushed into) the driving seat of health care commissioning and taking a lead on shaping local services.

Having influence, of course, also means having responsibilities and having to learn a range of new skills. It also means facing and overcoming new challenges. How does a general practitioner or a nurse, for example, balance the needs and demands of an individual patient with the pressures imposed by the finite resources available to a general practice or a community hospital? In the face of sometimes conflicting evidence on the effectiveness of treatments, or when the evidence is scanty and there is no evidence on cost-effectiveness between one intervention and another, how does one make the 'right' choice for a patient, or for groups of people who may have chronic and potentially life threatening problems?

The authors of this thoughtful book examine many of these challenges. In a rapidly changing environment they consider how general practice, particularly, and primary care in general, might be the focus for a re-orientated health care service for the 21st century. Information on effective practice is seen as a key component in this revolution. Improvements in access to evidence of effectiveness, better understanding of the means of taking evidence into practice, a recognition of the need to interpret evidence within the context of individual clinical circumstances: all of these developments are critical to enabling improvements in the quality of primary care.

So is the general practice and the primary health care team up to the task? By considering these issues within the context of rising public expectation, the authors identify a challenging agenda for primary care.

Allen Hutchinson
Chair, RCGP Quality Improvement Group
March 1997

1

An introduction to primary care

Health care systems are of three basic types: those which have no consistent structure, those which are based on a mixture of primary and specialist care, and those which are based on comprehensive primary care provision. It is generally observed that those systems which are based on comprehensive primary care have lower overall costs, less inequality in health and health care, less variation in the utilization of specialist care and a more even quality of care overall. These characteristics hold good at international, national and regional levels, but with decreasing certainty. Within those systems which already have comprehensive or limited primary care, the trend is towards greater empowerment of the primary care sector; the British NHS is an example of such a trend.

Primary care and the cost equation

In less structured systems, such as that operating in the United States, primary care development is seen as an important means of reducing the spiralling costs of health care. In these circumstances, the development of primary care is driven by the requirements of the agencies which fund health care, especially by employers through managed care organizations. The extremely high costs of these systems are due to the untrammelled efforts of specialists to commit resources towards the care of individual patients without reference to the cost to the patient or the underwriter, and too often with little attention paid to the clinical return on the investment. Primary care acts as a barrier to patient entry into the specialist health care arena and it reduces costs mainly by limiting access. It also shifts the balance of power within the health industry away from providers of care and towards the funders. This can be a two-edged sword as neither party has a monopoly on morality.

It is widely believed that the relatively low costs of health care in the United Kingdom are attributable to the effectiveness of primary care as a filter for specialist care. However, high hospitalization rates and long lengths of stay in the UK go some way towards wasting the spoils of primary care-based efficiency. In addition, primary care has never been managed in the UK; it operates as a state-funded private sector system with a mixture of local monopolies – especially in rural areas – and ill-informed local competition in urban settings. Wide variations are also observable in the competence of primary care as a filter for referrals to specialist care. These are explored further in Chapters 5 and 6.

The key ethical question is whether primary care affects overall costs by restricting access which is appropriate (unethical) or by limiting specialist care to that which is appropriate (ethical)? The probability is that the answer is a combination of the two but the moral high ground rests only with the limitation of care to that which is clinically appropriate and effective, regardless of the sector which provides it. It may be, therefore, that protocol-based care or, more properly, consistent evidence-based care is the criterion for high quality health care and that consistent, high quality primary care alone can create the right context for this.

Whence primary care?

The NHS has grown from a culture of widespread and accessible primary care dating back to the 1911 National Insurance Act (responsible for the widely held but mistaken belief that the NHS is paid for by National Insurance contributions) although comprehensiveness was a specific product of the creation of the NHS. In the USA, especially in the cities, comprehensive primary care does not operate in the same way as in the UK. Doctors work independently of the institutions of health care, there is greater use of specialist care and more extensive investigation and treatment of patients with conditions which would not be extensively pursued in other health systems. It is to control the costs of this clinical behaviour that managed care organizations, typically health maintenance organizations (HMOs), have introduced a tier of primary care physicians – often working to strict clinical protocols – to restrict inappropriate use of specialist and hospital care. By the standards operating in the UK even these protocols are liberal in their use of resources, but so great is the health care expenditure in the USA that the profit margins of managed care are embarrassingly large. This is not to say that there are not downward pressures on expenditure in the USA: indeed, in many respects they are greater than in the UK. It is the extraordinarily high baseline, the absence of ageism or sexism and the unremitting pursuit of the prolongation of life which increase health care costs. Some of these aspects are now playing a part in raising cost pressures on the NHS.

Whither primary care?

There are some similarities between the managed care model in the USA and the style of care now emerging in advanced fundholding and total purchasing schemes in seeking and occasionally producing the same scale of reductions in hospital and specialist care utilization. However, it is by no means clear that managed care is a good or even better model of health care than the ones it replaces. More economical it may be but does it deliver better health care for patients? In other words, does primary care succeed in this context merely because it acts as a filter for specialist care, saving patients from the excesses of experts, or does it offer an entirely different and better model of care overall, a holistic and patient-based approach to health care and a sound foundation for the introduction of evidence-based medicine?

The hypothesis in favour of primary care as the base for all health care assumes that the merits of holism and unification of health care exceed the added value of ultimate specialization. In this model, the treatment of the individual and their family is considered to be of greater importance than the pursuit of the last fragment of health gain for a specific disease. The evidence base to support this approach is strictly limited but it has become the political norm in the UK and commands much support with the general public. There remains a view, however, that patients should be treated by specialists and that the role of the generalist is to refer to the right specialty.

The global context

The World Health Organization (WHO), in its espoused global strategy for health – widely misquoted but known as 'Health for All' – adopted the principles of the Alma Ata declaration.[1] This was the product of an international conference on primary care as the basis for achieving its goals worldwide. Due partly to the difficulties of translating strategic goals into scores of different languages and the need to satisfy widely varying national interests, it is not altogether clear that the WHO description of primary care equates to the current structure and role of primary care in the NHS.

Box 1.1: Section V of the Alma Ata declaration

Governments have a responsibility for the health of their people which can be fulfilled only by the provision of adequate health and social measures. A main social target of governments, international organizations and the whole world community in the coming decades should be the attainment by all peoples of the world by the year 2000 of a level of health that will permit them to lead a socially and economically productive life. Primary health care is the key to attaining this target as part of development in the spirit of social justice.

Given the economic context outlined above, it is arguable that any global strategy for health which was not based on primary care would not be universally attainable and, therefore, the world had no alternative but to adopt primary care as the main vehicle for achieving health for all. However, to argue so would be to underestimate the strengths of primary care as a way of delivering health care. It is, for example, the only way to ensure comprehensiveness, a principle enshrined in both the title and pro-gramme of Health for All. It is also a necessary component of any system which sets out to avoid or reduce iatrogenic disease by the avoidance of

---

Box 1.2: Section VI of the Alma Ata declaration[1]

Primary health care is essential health care based on practical, scientifically sound and socially acceptable methods and technology, made universally acces-sible to individuals and families in the community through their full participa-tion and at a cost that the community and country can afford to maintain at every stage of their development in the spirit of self-reliance and self-determination. It forms an integral part both of the country's health system, of which it is the central function and main focus, and of the overall social and economic development of the community. It is the first level of contact of individuals, the family and community with the national health system, bringing health care as close as possible to where people live and work, and constitutes the first element of a continuing health care process.

---

inappropriate specialist care. Comprehensive primary care is almost certainly the best way, indeed a prerequisite, for reducing inequalities in health between nations and between peoples within nations – a key goal of all Health for All strategies and now recognized in the UK's Health of the Nation strategy.

The extracts from the Alma Ata declaration (Boxes 1.1 and 1.2) demonstrate how far-sighted the world's leaders were almost 20 years ago and how far the so-called developed countries have to go in achieving the basic infrastructure of a fair health care system.

We may justifiably conclude that comprehensive primary care is the core component of any strategy for equality in health care and a major factor in securing equality in health experience also. This essentially socialist goal is at odds with the use of primary care for economic gain and the introduction of competitive principles and disciplines into the health systems of the UK and USA during the last decade. What is less clear is how a primary care-based service affects the quality of care overall. The avoidance of excesses of specialization is a generally positive aspect but it is uncertain that the primary care service provides substitution of proven and sufficient quality in a technical sense. The adoption of primary care by governments and other funders of health care to reduce costs and improve coverage requires the quality question to be answered positively for their strategies to be blessed with morality. So long as there is an absence of systems to assure the quality of primary care provision, primary care can be all things to all people!

The primary care vision

The specialty of public health medicine often claims to be the discipline which acts as the physician for populations. In practice, it operates at some distance from populations and although general practices function at a smaller population level and do not often possess all the skills required for analysis of population health, they are closer to the real life of communities and are able to add the intangible perspectives of community observation to the analytical facts of health. It is fair to argue, therefore, that primary care is in a unique position to view all aspects of health care in the wider context at practice population level, and that public health intelligence is the sum of primary care knowledge.

Specialists who work mainly in hospital, with the increasing exclusion of general paediatricians, general psychiatrists and physicians in elderly medicine, have a very limited view of life. Their work is dominated by a small number of common conditions, often no more than four or five, and a larger group of rare conditions of relevance to individuals but scarcely to populations. Their understanding of how their patients live is extremely restricted and, often, of little interest to them. General practice can be regarded as the opposite of this analysis with the exception that a high proportion of clinical contacts, perhaps 30%, have a mental health component, albeit with aetiological origins in the micro-environment and especially the home.

The other group of people who would like to think that they understand the world is politicians. They are, after all, elected to represent the whole electorate; one can forgive them for mistakenly believing that they know what the people think. Politicians are, so far as health is concerned, pursuing the avoidance of (political) risks and problems. These occur mostly in terms of overall funding, patient rights (e.g. equality of access) and isolated aspects of specialist care such as the potential homicidal behaviour of severely mentally ill patients. General practice, as the source of most NHS provision, has not often entered into their consciousness unless there has been a professional dispute or a crisis of confidence.

One must conclude, therefore, that only primary care professionals, and general medical practitioners in particular, are able to visualize the life and needs of communities and that more credence needs to be given to primary care as a source of knowledge about health development needs.

Primary care policy

Despite the central importance of primary care to the ethos and practice of the NHS, and its value in controlling overall costs of health care to the government, health policy pays relatively little credence to primary care interests. This is not just a characteristic of the post-1979 era with its emphasis on customer empowerment and cost reductions, it applies throughout the history of the NHS. From time to time, general practitioners reassert themselves and secure a better deal for those working in the primary care sector but, until the reforms of the early 1990s, there was no attempt by politicians to use primary care as the main vehicle for change.

The reason for the relatively limited impact which primary care has on policy has more to do with power structures in the medical profession than with government or civil service intent; indeed, generalists are more highly rated than specialists in the civil service generally. In the professions, specialization gives power through knowledge and power attracts the attention of politicians.

Both government and the public tend to take general medical practice for granted: it is the visible face of the health service and almost all people are familiar with it as regular users. Primary care, dominated as it is by the structure of medical practice, is not seen as a problem by government. The staff are not usually government employees and there are well-established complaints systems which run smoothly and are probably underused. Recent revision of these systems is not the result of clear evidence of their failure but is indicative of the proposed empowerment of the users of all public services, including those provided by the professions.

Medical specialists have a different view of primary care. They regard generalists with some disdain, unless the practitioners do some work directly for them, and regard expertise as essential for competent practice. They see general practice as a problem due to the lack of consistency and, in some cases, a shortage of clinical competence and confidence. Conversely, and sometimes perversely, general practitioners see the specialist community as a problem, taking over clinical responsibility when only an opinion is sought, using investigative and treatment resources excessively and failing to communicate effectively with patients, with each other and with themselves. The inability of many specialists to treat patients holistically is a serious failure in terms of the ethos of general practice and, as with the competence of general practitioners, not all specialists are regarded as equal. Indeed, there is no more reason to assume a consistency of quality or opinion in specialist care than one is likely to find in general practice in most of the country.

This somewhat sordid stand-off between branches of the same profession is not one which politicians, either party or professional, wish to get entwined with. They concentrate instead on the visible and unavoidable problems of health care: lack of capital and estate development needs, rising costs, new clinical technologies, waiting times for treatment, communicable disease and gross neglect. On these issues, it is thought, all stakeholders can unite; although even here stark differences of perception can emerge in, say, the importance of waiting times.

A further confounding variable, the result of gender equality legislation of the 1960s, is the increasing trend for medical marriage partnerships with one marriage partner in primary care and the other employed as a hospital specialist. This is leading to a wider understanding of the respective roles, values and strengths of the two sectors although many of the players are relatively young and not yet opinion leaders. The recent staffing crisis in general practice is a crisis amongst men; recruitment of women into general practice has held up well.

The main thrust of government policy on health has tended to avoid primary care explicitly for many years although several mainstream policies, such as community care for the elderly and mentally ill and day-case surgery, have had an unquantified and, at best, indirectly resourced impact on primary care practice. Recent initiatives by the UK government in reforming the NHS appear to have rediscovered primary care as an important agent of change. However, the focus of most of these changes, such as fundholding, is the role which general practice can play in changing the style and cost of specialist care. The consequential changes in investment in primary care are seen as a by-product of fundholding rather than a specific set of goals.

What is happening to primary care?

There are many definitions of primary care, all of them right for some. The common features of primary care are that it is a place where care is provided and it is not hospital. Primary care, as its name implies, deals with first contacts between patients and health services. We could also add that it is multidisciplinary in nature, is relatively non-invasive and provides continuity over long periods of time. General medical practice, the fundamental core of primary care, is not synonymous with this definition of primary care. It is normally unidisciplinary and is concerned with a limited range of specific clinical services.

Returning to the global context, Box 1.3 summarizes the attempt in the Alma Ata declaration to define primary health care. This clearly places primary care at the heart of a nation's infrastructure and reflects a country's culture and values. The WHO approach is far ahead of its time in terms of user empowerment and the broad tapestry of public health approaches to the pressures of modern living. It also seeks to demedicalize the basis of primary care, which has been more easily achieved in developing countries than in developed societies with medically led services which have been long established.

One of the most important changes currently occurring is a blurring of the boundary between hospital and primary care. The direction of drift is almost wholly towards primary care as the activities and staff involved in hospital out-patients become more mobile and the principles of the fundholding scheme encourage their mobility. It is probable that these changes would have commenced without the reforms of the NHS and the introduction of fundholding simply because the technical capacity to investigate

> **Box 1.3: Adapted from Section VII of the Alma Ata declaration[1]**
>
> Primary health care:
>
> - reflects economic conditions and political characteristics of the country
> - is based on the results of biomedical and health services research
> - provides promotive, preventive, curative and rehabilitative services
> - includes education concerning prevention; an adequate supply of safe water; promotion of proper nutrition
> - includes maternal and child health, including family planning, immunization against infectious diseases, treatment of common disease and injuries
> - involves all related sectors, in particular agriculture, animal husbandry, food, industry, education, housing, public works, communications
> - promotes maximum community and individual self-reliance in the planning, organization, operation and control of primary health care
> - should be sustained by integrated, functional referral systems, leading to the progressive improvement of comprehensive health care for all, and giving priority to those most in need
> - relies on health workers, including physicians, nurses, midwives, auxiliaries and community workers, as well as traditional practitioners as needed, to work as a health team

and assess outside hospital is now widespread and the increasing number of professional staff enables them to increase their peripatetic style.

In the longer term, it is likely that most out-patient assessment and most investigation can be conducted outside a formal hospital setting and therefore within the potential control of primary care. There are also examples in leading-edge fundholding practices and total purchasing schemes of general practitioner hospitals developing as part of the practice, and the development of operating capacity in or close to primary care settings.

To support these changes, general practice partnerships are starting to become multidisciplinary and the stable base of the NHS, the dependable primary care taken for granted by all, is undergoing significant, rapid, and therefore unpredictable change.

During the last five years, more than half of all practices have adopted fundholding responsibilities, making explicit their long-standing ability to commit resources and supported by rules which enable them to move resources from one sector of health care to another. Their own prescribing has come under closer supervision and major progress has been made in reducing variation and improving efficient prescribing practices. This has been assisted by financial incentives for fundholders and, later, for non-fundholding practices too. Practices have made new strides in developing health promotion packages and chronic disease management for people with diabetes and asthma; and in providing routine surveillance for elderly people and for middle-aged people at risk of ischaemic heart disease. The government has made specific investment in research and development in primary care, making it the first priority for research infrastructure investment by establishing a national research centre based in Manchester, Salford and York Universities.[2] Finally, the profession's long-standing commitment to provide 24-hour cover for its patients has been restructured to reduce the burden on individual practitioners and to improve the coverage of care; this move is a response to dramatic increases in the demand for night-time care, sometimes for trivial reasons.

The traffic is not, however, all in one direction. There is growing evidence from the hospital service that general practitioners are increasingly likely to refer patients to specialist care. Box 1.4 summarizes the key shifts in services between the sectors.

Box 1.4: Service shifts between primary and secondary care

From primary care:

- rising emergency admissions

- increasing elective referrals

- rising A&E attendances

From secondary care:

- management of common chronic disease, e.g. asthma, diabetes, hypertension

- near patient testing

- practice-based consultant clinics

- earlier hospital discharges

- home/nursing home-based continuing care

Is general practice changing too?

The NHS reforms of the 1990s purport to introduce competitiveness into the NHS. As all doctors know, competitiveness is second nature to members of the medical profession: it is required to qualify in medicine, to enter specialist or general practice training and to obtain a career post or partnership. It did not require political action to create competitiveness in medicine.

The reforms of the NHS implemented from 1991 onwards, and the preceding reform of the general practitioners' contract, encouraged competitive behaviour within practice. Increasing the proportion of practice income which is linked to patient numbers pushed practices to become attractive to patients where alternative practices were available. The funding arrangements for hospital care, and particularly the innovation from fundholders, helped to exaggerate the competitiveness in the NHS. The general, though not universal, response will be a rise in standards of customer care in the practice. Unfortunately for practices, it is almost certain that patient expectations will rise faster than the capacity of practices to meet them. Although there are some examples of organizational competitiveness in the new NHS, the creed is mainly confined to a relatively few individuals and the intrinsic beliefs in the values of collectivism have persisted amongst the majority of professional staff.

The policy-drivers

This book is primarily concerned with the implementation of the NHS research and development (R&D) strategy through the medium of primary care. The context in which this is promoted includes the primary care-based purchasing structure but is not confined to those practices involved in fundholding. The culture of primary care has changed across the board – faster in some leading purchasers it is true – but no practice has been untouched by the changes of the early 1990s.

The R&D strategy was a response by the government to criticism from the House of Lords Select Committee on Science and Technology about the way in which it funded and managed health-related research.[3] Of particular concern to their Lordships was the failure of successive governments to address the research needs of public health and operational systems for health care delivery, a field known generically as 'health services research'.[4]

Not only did the response create a new national leadership post of Director of Research and Development, held for the first five years by Professor Sir Michael Peckham, but it led to the internalization of research management into the NHS. Partly because the aforementioned failures had been achieved by the Department of Health's own staff, and partly because a new culture of proximity of research to management was sought, the strategy was developed and achieved in close partnership with those parts of the NHS which the Department of Health recognized, i.e. regional health authorities (RHAs). While RHAs were regarded as central bur-eaucracy by most NHS staff, to the Department they were operational NHS.

During the early 1990s three major changes occurred: first, the research and development genre developed within the NHS; second, the power and influence of primary care grew; third, RHAs were abolished and their func-tions were transferred either to the new district health authorities (DHAs) or to new, but small, regional offices of the NHS Executive.

The characteristics of the second of these changes is widely discussed throughout this book, but the others deserve greater mention here. The adoption of an R&D strategy for the NHS was without political discord at a time when the NHS was a major political battleground and, as in all wars, truth was the first victim. So morally robust was the research agenda that no public opposition was countenanced towards the strategy although there were many doubters in private amongst both the medical profession and the research community. The active management of the strategy through RHAs sought to secure the ownership of both clinicians and managers and, to some extent, overcame professional doubts. The strategy was system-atically extended to involve other professions and specifically to focus on primary care, the subject of the largest single research infrastructure in-vestment by the Department of Health in its history. With hindsight, how-ever, this honeymoon period was founded on a basic lack of understanding of the goals of the R&D strategy and the ways in which it would affect the working of different stakeholders.

While the R&D strategy was bedding into the NHS as we all knew it, forces were at work to destabilize the management arrangements yet again. This time, and for the first time since the creation of the NHS, it was the regional tier which was targeted rather than the operational services. The RHAs had been responsible for implementing the 1991 reforms. By 1993/ 94, that task was all but complete and their own demise was planned. The functions and manpower review (FMR)[5] of the NHS Executive and RHAs which followed exposed serious divisions within the NHS Executive, especially between the medical division and the R&D division.

The R&D information initiative was directed to disseminate the results of reliable research, existing and new, which would have an impact on practice in the NHS. Various structural components of this initiative were established, including the highly praised Cochrane Collaboration – an international partnership which maintained overviews of the results of randomized controlled trials for clinical conditions – and the Centre for Reviews and Dissemination, which was concerned more with evidence which could be used by purchasers of health care. These systems were established by 1993 when the medical division of the NHS Executive decided to issue its own proposals for implementing changes in clinical practice, an initiative it titled 'clinical effectiveness'. This consisted of the distribution by circular[6] of a list of clinical guidelines for common though not mainstream conditions, confined almost exclusively to hospital care, and dismissed by all objective observers as opinion-based rather than evidence-based. A further exercise the following year was only marginally better conducted. This behaviour was symptomatic of a power battle within the NHS Executive between the public health-led medical division and the R&D division. The final result of the FMR was a victory on points for R&D with both disciplines having Board-level status within the national and regional Executive Board arrangements.

The paradigm shift takes hold

The NHS has a set of values and principles which are all its own. They are held in common and taken for granted throughout the organization. Central to the NHS paradigm has been the principle of clinical freedom, defined extensively in jocular terms but basically meaning that clinical professionals are free to do the wrong things so long as they did not intend to harm the patient. The other cardinal feature of the NHS paradigm was the collectivism of the service as a whole. This the reforms have sought to destroy and to replace with a passion for competition, but with only limited success.

Paradigms have been blown apart in many industries, services and professions since the Thatcherite reforms took root in the early 1980s, but there had been relatively little impact on the NHS until the 1991 reforms. Although the NHS trusts have certainly responded to the new scenario, and the NHS R&D strategy heralds a fundamental change in attitudes to clinical freedom, the dominant force in changing the paradigm of the NHS is the behaviour of general practices. They are not alone, however, as growing public questioning also has a role in diverting the NHS into new patterns of response.

It could be argued that even without the reforms public attitudes would eventually have driven through changes in service style and professional attitudes, but it would have taken much longer to take hold. The principal changes which can be anticipated during the next decade include reduced variation in clinical practices, reduced tolerance by the whole population of waiting for care, public unwillingness to accept the inevitability of death and the failure of health care, a relative and gradual fall in professional prestige (in common with other professions), increasingly open competitive behaviour and an increasingly mixed economy for health care.

The last of these, the growing privately insured population and the increasing strength and flexibility of the private sector, is substantially dependent on the confidence of general practitioners, the wealth of the community and the flexibility of insurers for it to prosper. Some practices may prefer to offer higher quality care within their own premises rather than sending patients into privately owned institutions. The future structure of the private sector may owe more to primary care innovation than can currently be imagined.

The health agendas which have managed to avoid the bitter political disputes of the last decade are relatively few in number. Foremost amongst them is the growing emphasis on evidence-based health care with the objectives both of reducing unjustified variation in clinical practice (and costs) and improving the outcome of clinical care. Not all evidence-based health care will cost less: there is growing evidence that the health care provided in the UK is nihilistic by international standards and that clinically effective care will cost more initially. Nonetheless, the focus on evidence from reliable research and the implementation of effective clinical care will be popular facets of the future health care system in all developed nations.

A second emerging health agenda which will persist for the foreseeable future is concern over variations or inequalities in health. The role of health care in reducing inequalities is unclear and is almost certainly less than other factors such as wealth, education, employment and personal behaviour such as smoking tobacco and abuse of alcohol. However, equalizing access to health care when needs exist is a goal which no developed nation has achieved. Clinical effectiveness is independent of class, creed or culture and must form the basis of any policy of equalizing care for needs.

Primary care, and especially primary medical care, holds the key to the kingdom of success in these astonishingly ambitious health goals. The future of the NHS depends on the willingness and capacity of primary care to rise to the challenge. Clinically effective practice is at the heart of the future of health care.

References

1 World Health Organization (1978) *Health for All* (the Alma Ata declaration) WHO, Copenhagen.
2 Annual report of the National Centre for Primary Care Research, University of Manchester (1996).
3 House of Lords Select Committee on Science and Technology (1988) *Priorities in Medical Research.* HMSO, London.
4 Peckham M (1991) *Research for Health.* Department of Health, London.
5 NHS Executive (1994) *Managing the New NHS. Functions and Responsibilities in the New NHS.* NHSE, Leeds.
6 NHS Management Executive (1993) *Improving Clinical Effectiveness* (EL(93)115). NHSME, Leeds.

2

A primary care-led NHS in the modern world

The comprehensive system of primary medical care, which underpins service equality and access, is the most enduring and unique characteristic of the NHS. The creation of the NHS in 1948 consisted of two key changes: the nationalization of the hospitals (previously a mixture of voluntary hospitals and local authority-run general and specialist hospitals and asylums) and the introduction of a contract between general medical practitioners and the government. The principal characteristic of this contract was the universal right of a patient to have their own doctor and the right of the doctor to be rewarded financially by the government. Until then, a range of schemes had operated providing primary care for those in employment and their families but with a proportion of the population excluded and seeking care from other, less convenient and impersonal, public provision such as dispensaries, or effectively being denied care because of unaffordability.

The rights of every citizen to have their own doctor and to receive appropriate medical care free at the point of delivery were unique at the time and, although other systems have improved upon the post-war British innovation, these basic principles remain largely intact.

The independent contractor

The contractual relationship between general practitioners and the government allows the doctors to be self-employed and/or in partnership and to receive payment from the Department of Health in exchange for an agreed set of services and commitments. The rules covering this arrangement are agreed between the government and the General Medical Services Committee of the British Medical Association and contained within the Statement of Fees and Allowances, commonly known as the 'Red Book'.[1] This arrangement has been administered by local committees since 1948: Executive Councils from 1948–74, by Family Practitioner Committees from 1974–89 (initially as committees of area health authorities and district health authorities; from 1985 as authorities in their own right), and by the renamed and restructured family health services authorities (FHSAs) since 1989. These functions transferred to the new district health authorities in 1996.[2] At no time throughout the history of the NHS has there been any attempt to manage the provision of primary health care delivered by general practitioners.

The 'Red Book' of rules describes in detail what is expected of doctors in terms of their commitment of time, their responsibilities to patients and what they are entitled to receive payment for. It does not lay down standards of medical practice nor does it enable or encourage critical examination of clinical performance. There is no quality assurance system nor the framework for peer review. Such matters have always been too contentious for either politicians or the profession to attempt to address systematically – until now, perhaps.

The impact of reform

Since 1990, many reforms have been imposed upon the NHS and primary medical care in particular. Of most importance were the implications of the two White Papers of 1988 and 1989, 'Promoting Better Health'[3] and 'Working for Patients'.[4] These introduced a new contract for general medical practitioners with more detail about the tasks they were expected to perform as part of their contractual commitment; professional review of their prescribing practices by a medical professional adviser to the FHSA (and later a pharmaceutical adviser); the introduction of indicative prescribing amounts for practices (effectively an average prescribing budget based on weighted populations); introducing payment for achieving practice population targets for immunization and cervical cytology uptake – rewarding success but accentuating failure; new payments for health promotion activity – some of which was, and remains, branded as pointless – and clinical audit to monitor work for diabetics and asthma sufferers; and, most divisive of all, the option for larger practices of becoming fundholders and purchasing some hospital and community services direct from specialist hospital providers.

The so-called 'GP fundholders', originally described as 'budget holders' in the White Paper 'Working for Patients',[5] had to be large practices (over 11 000 patients, though by the time of the first wave of fundholding this had been reduced to 9000 and has subsequently been reduced further), which were effectively and successfully computerized and which had the will and capacity to manage relatively large amounts of public money. Included in the 'fund' were all the staff costs associated with their own practice, which were paid for by the NHS under the 'Red Book' terms and conditions, together with all the costs of drugs prescribed by partners of the practice and their staff and subsequently dispensed. In addition, a sum of money was transferred from health authorities to cover the cost of hospital and community services which until then the practice purchased from the NHS. The range of services covered by this arrangement increased in each year of the scheme but always included all out-patient care, most investigations and most elective surgery. Community nursing and other services were added later. By the mid-1990s, average fundholders purchased 20% of all services for their practice population, worth almost £2 million for the average fundholding practice and constituting the largest element of the fund.[6] The growth in the fundholding scheme is catalogued in Box 2.1.[6,7]

The purchasing and drug elements of the fund were based initially on past practice but gradual moves were made by health authorities towards fair-share budgets based on populations adjusted for age and sex using nationally adopted formulae. Fundholders were able to buy the services they wanted from any provider, private or NHS, and could even provide some themselves.

Most fundholding practices found it relatively easy to save money on both prescribing costs (by increasing their generic prescribing, for example) and the use of hospital services by reducing referrals or making arrangements in the practice for patients to be seen by specialists. The rules of the fundholding scheme allowed them to invest these surpluses in facilities or services which benefited their patients and many new practice premises were built, or existing buildings improved, as a result. The whole scheme was voluntary – although peer and political pressure was a significant factor in creating volunteers – and lessons on how to maximize practice benefits were quickly learned. For example, fundholders constrained prescribing costs more quickly and effectively than other practices[8] and they retained the financial savings.

These changes had profound effects upon the whole NHS but the impact on primary care was explosive. Not only was the profession divided into pro- and anti-fundholder camps, mainly though not entirely on political lines initially, but practices actively competed to be more innovative with other peoples' money. The fundholding initiative was regarded as the jewel in the crown of the government's highly unpopular reform programme. As well as stimulating changes in the way hospital services were delivered, the initiative forced general practitioners and hospital consultants to talk to

Box 2.1: Developments in the fundholding scheme[6,7]

General practitioner fundholding:

- Introduced by NHS and Community Care Act 1990.

- GPs who volunteer for the scheme receive a budget to cover the costs of some hospital and community services, prescriptions for drugs and the salaries of non-medical practice staff.

- The average standard fundholding practice has a budget of £1.7 million (1994/95 figures). This translates to £140–£170 per patient for the majority of practices but there is a threefold variation between extremes.

- Fundholding is less common in deprived areas; there are more GP training practices in fundholding.

- Fundholders purchase about 20% of their patients' hospital and community healthcare by value – mainly services that are planned in advance rather than emergencies.

- From their fund, GPs spend 29% on planned operations, 6% on mental health and learning disabilities, 16% on community nursing, 6% on pathology and X-ray, 40% on surgical and medical outpatients, and 3% on direct access, e.g. physiotherapy.

- Practices needed a minimum of 9000 patients to be eligible for the first wave of fundholding in 1991. Over the next five years the regulations governing the scheme changed and in 1996 practices with 5000 patients were eligible to join. Over the same period the lists of services that fundholders can purchase lengthened.

- Community fundholding allows practices with as few as 3000 patients to purchase community health services, drugs and practice staff, but not hospital services. Practices with fewer than 5000 patients can also form a consortium with one or more other practices to participate in standard fundholding.

- In 1996 more than 50% of the population were registered with a fundholding practice.

- Up to the end of 1994/95 fundholding practices had received £232 million to cover the costs of staff, equipment and computers in managing fundholding. In addition there are new transaction costs in hospitals and health authorities. The £206 million efficiency savings made by fundholders over the same period do not match these costs. Are quality improvements made by fundholders tipping the balance in favour of fundholding? Are these setup costs which will, over time, be outweighed by continuing, and perhaps increasing, efficiency savings?

each other in a way which had never been achieved, that is on equal terms. The benefits of this dialogue proved the most significant and relevant in the early years of the reformed NHS. Eventually, many professional objections to fundholding were overcome or, more commonly, set aside, as entry criteria to the scheme were relaxed and more practices wanted to avail themselves of the dialogue on equal terms with hospital colleagues, though divisions in the profession remained. By 1995, a majority of general practitioners were involved in fundholding and many were looking towards the next development, the purchasing of all specialist health care by primary care practitioners.

Continuing reform

Late in 1994, the government published a pamphlet describing the future in terms of a primary care-led NHS.[9] This proposed a range of extensions to the fundholding scheme, making it clear that this was the right, proper and normal way for general practice to develop. The most dramatic extension of the scheme built on a small number of unevaluated pilot studies in which all health services for a practice population, groups of practices or a defined geographical area were purchased by a Board of general practitioners acting on behalf of the district health authority. Unlike standard fundholding, the additional resources would remain in the ownership of the health authorities and surpluses could not be used directly by the practices involved. These total purchasing projects were open to fundholders, non-fundholders or a mixture, but practices or the equivalent had to demonstrate their competence with NHS funds and the intended benefits of the proposed purchasing arrangements. By 1996, about 5% of the population was covered by these schemes and over 50% by some form of fundholding.

The accompanying information to the pamphlet[9] suggested that the government's intended meaning of 'a primary care-led NHS' referred specifically to primary care leadership of the purchasing of secondary care, a process which was already well advanced. A draft accountability framework for general practitioners involved in this work was issued shortly afterwards. Although never publicly acknowledged, a more exciting and threatening possibility existed in terms of extending the accountability of general practitioners beyond that of their purchasing decisions as fundholders and to include their own provision of primary care services.

Since the introduction of the fundholding scheme in 1991, participating practices have been held to account for their purchasing decisions in health terms and for financial management of the totality of funds made available to them (including their own prescribing and practice costs). This accountability was formally to the regional tier of management in the NHS (the regional health authority) although normally exercised on the RHA's behalf by the local family health services' authority. The extension of the scheme to the purchasing of all health services had a different structure, the purchasing schemes being part of the district health authority's function. Accountability rested at that level, with the authority accountable for the totality of its purchasing, including that done on its behalf by general practitioners. With the abolition of RHAs in 1996, the role of DHAs in primary care development and management rose in importance and the accountability of fundholders became more local in nature. The creation of the new district health authorities absorbing the previous functions of both DHAs and FHSAs also contributed to the new environment for the developing of primary care-led purchasing and established primary care (development and management) as their main area of responsibility.

There are other interpretations of the meaning of a primary care-led NHS. At one end of the spectrum is the prospect of subcontracting all purchasing of hospital and community health services to primary care, both enabling a major disinvestment from the bureaucracy of health authorities and introducing the notion of privatizing the purchasing of health care, general practitioners being, strictly speaking, private sector partnerships. Such ideas have never been publicly espoused by Ministers, but senior government advisers have acknowledged the political attractiveness of the privatization of purchasing (although the evidence from fundholding is that the transaction costs of devolved purchasing are much higher than those of health authorities). Given the unpleasant reality that the most basic principle of the public service is the centralization of control and the delegation of blame, it is unlikely that such a move would prove to be in the interests of primary care. At the other extreme, it is possible to envisage, in the extension of primary care purchasing, the end of the independence of primary care contractors. With primary care purchasers accountable to district health authorities for their purchasing decisions, why should they not also be made accountable for the services they provide in primary care? After all, the large majority of clinical care is provided mainly or wholly within the primary care setting: how can accountability for the whole service be extended without addressing primary care provision? Furthermore, as primary care purchasing developed alongside the development of primary care provision, it becomes increasingly difficult to draw clear boundaries between the definitions of primary and secondary care.

The drive for reform continued with the publication of yet another White Paper in 1996 entitled 'Choice and Opportunity'.[10] Unlike previous reforms, this specifically addressed the structure of primary care provision, promoted the idea of pilot projects with escape clauses and commands a degree of support, though not universal, of all political parties and the medical profession. The proposals in 'Choice and Opportunity' provided the first potential break in the 1948 model of primary care, including the possibility of directly employed practitioners and the merger of primary and secondary care provision through trusts. At the time of writing, it is unclear how quickly these changes will be implemented but the absence of any fierce opposition suggests that choices and opportunities will indeed be made and taken.

The political objectives of reform

The NHS reforms had two main components: the introduction of market disciplines into the use of resources in the NHS; and the creation of independent organizations, known as NHS trusts, within the NHS but with the structure of quasi-private health care organizations and using a financial regime which ensured their competing on equal terms with health care providers wholly within the private sector. The objectives of reform included improved efficiency of the service and reflection of the needs and desires of patients more effectively. There was also a clear steer towards increasing the role and size of the private sector through tax relief on health insurance premiums for the elderly and encouraging private/public sector partnerships and competition.

The role of the fundholding scheme in this scenario was twofold. First, it was thought unlikely that health authorities would be effective purchasers, at least in the first instance, and fundholders were looked to as stimulators of the market and to lead innovation in purchasing in the short term. Second, it was considered probable that fundholders would shift some work from the NHS trusts to private providers, thus helping to expand the private health sector overall, eventually to shift the balance of the market sufficiently for privatization of the whole service to be considered both feasible and acceptable to the public. Setting aside the last point, it is fair to argue that fundholding delivered to some extent on both these roles although analyses of the benefits of fundholding in the mid-1990s tended to be rather downbeat. In particular, it was felt that the large majority of fundholders had not done enough to improve health care, merely spending slightly less on drug costs or fruitless out-patient consultations and more on their own premises.[6] Perversely, it appears likely that health authorities were as attentive learners of the tricks of purchasing from leading-edge fundholders as were any new practices entering the scheme, and that the clear advantage which fundholders started with was reduced over time. The real value of fundholding may therefore have been the shift in power between consultants and general practitioners.

The need for leadership

Both the possible extension of primary care accountability and the sense that general practitioners were being used to achieve political goals on which they had not been consulted would be an alarming prospect for the Luddite great and good who, through the British Medical Association, purport to represent the profession in its dealings with government. However, there is reason to believe that many leading practitioners in the purchasing field recognized clearly enough the extended implications of the changes taking place and in which they were actively participating. However, the professions have long held the mistaken belief that they can use others in government to help pursue their own ends while it suits them and then break the relationship when they choose. The German middle classes thought the same about Adolf Hitler!

It is unlikely to be a rapid move towards primary care accountability for primary care provision: the sensitivities and the risks are too great for it to be rushed. But accountability of the professions, in all walks of life, is an inevitable consequence of the increasing empowerment of the population – albeit shot through with individualistic consumerism, a popular movement which cannot be reversed within our democracy and is not dependent on a particular political party being in power. Medicine will face up to this reality with the same pain that other leading professions are experiencing. The primary care-led NHS may well prove to be no more than a step towards user empowerment and a patient-led NHS in the fullness of time.

How great a change will it make for the population served by general medical practitioners if they are held accountable for the services they provide? The first significant difference will be a greater openness about what they should be doing, where, when, whether and how. Until now, government policies on health, such as the Health of the Nation strategy,[11] have largely passed by primary care without affecting it, despite the fact that the target areas cover about half of all their work (Box 2.2). Accountable

---

Box 2.2: Health of the Nation target areas

1 Coronary heart disease and stroke
   smoking
   diet and nutrition
   blood pressure

2 Cancers
   breast
   cervical
   lung
   skin

3 Mental illness
   health and social functioning of mentally ill people
   suicides
   suicide amongst seriously mentally ill people

4 HIV/AIDS and sexual health
   gonorrhoea
   conceptions under 16 years
   drug misusers sharing injecting equipment

5 Accidents
   death rate under 15 years
   death rate aged 15–24 years
   death rate over 65 years

---

general practitioners are brought into the fold of responsibility for delivering services and achieving targets. This is not so new because general practitioners have long participated in national immunization programmes but only since 1990 have population targets been defined and achieved and success rewarded.

General practitioners have a particular role to play in helping to achieve Health of the Nation targets for ischaemic heart disease and stroke through the effective identification and treatment of hypertension, advice on the cessation of smoking and possibly the identification and management of risk through reducing high cholesterol levels. They also play a key role in reducing the incidence of cervical cancer through ensuring the maximum possible uptake of screening. Improving mental health through better management of mild and moderate mental ill health and participating in joint management of the severely mentally ill and action on lung cancer through the reduction in smoking are also necessary components of high quality primary care. Yet these laudable goals were not addressed specifically to primary care in the first instance and the advice industry which the Department of Health has inflicted on the NHS, following the publication of the Health of the Nation, has still not addressed the central role of primary care in achieving success.

A new primacy for primary care

The NHS has largely failed to understand primary care until now and the jury remains out on its current performance. A new NHS based on primary care leadership is more than a delegation of blame to general practitioners: it requires a shared ownership of complex problems and a commitment from the government and its health authorities to view the health service through the eyes of primary care rather than through the distorted vision of hospital specialists. The investment in health care should follow patients' clinical needs rather than professional aspirations. For primary care this means a continuation of the increase in its influence, a growing role in purchasing secondary care but also greater accountability for the cost and quality of its own contribution to the totality of health care. Primary care is also well placed to exert greater accountability on specialist services, a fact which effective fundholders are now using with devastating effect.

The politics of primary care

Primary care is a health service setting: it is not synonymous with general medical practice but the latter is the dominant force in primary care provision. The pre-eminence of medicine is due largely to two factors: first, it is through medical practice that most primary care is delivered; second, the structure of the NHS depends mainly on where the doctors are and all else is organized around them. Usually, other staff working in the primary care sector are employed by medical practices: increasingly so as fundholding and other reforms have led to the internalization of more community care services into practices. There are also significant unmet opportunities for enhancing the framework, quality and efficiency of primary care by extending its scope into pharmacology, etc.

One of the dominant features of general practice is the ownership of the premises and the purchase of partnership rights. The cost-rent scheme, which has improved the ease and affordability of premises development, is only available to medical practice partnerships. In general, only the doctors have the income and security required to enter into such risky and long-term investments. This has helped to maintain the medical dominance of primary care and, as the fundholding scheme has increased the availability of re-sources to invest in premises, the closed shop for partnerships has been sustained, though not absolutely. Some practices have salaried partners who belong to other professions such as nursing and practice management. Furthermore, with the growth of the primary care sector and its expansion into areas of work previously limited to hospitals, medicine is conceivably threatened with becoming a minority profession in primary care at some time in the foreseeable future.

It is quite unclear at the present time how primary care will evolve during the next decade. It is likely that clinical management issues around the effect-ive treatment of patients will become more explicit and that the wide varia-tions currently observed in practice, especially in the proportion of patients referred to specialists, will reduce. The extent to which general practice will remain a closed shop for doctors is uncertain but, if trends elsewhere are followed, more multidisciplinary involvement is likely. As pay structures in general become less centralized, it is also possible that full partnerships, especially for managers in primary care, are possible. The recent changes in out-of-hours cover and responsibility could be paradigm shifting in nature, allowing unimaginable flexibility in local arrangements if the 1990 contract becomes subject to locally agreed amendments and, as offered in 'Choice and Opportunity', the commissioning of primary care becomes a flexible option.

Medical politics

General practitioners form the single largest group within the medical profession in the UK, though this is not the case in many other countries. More than one-third of all working doctors are engaged in general practice and there are far more GP principals (28 000) than there are hospital special-ists (21 000). However, the prestige of specialists, both within the profession and in the eyes of the general public, has greatly exceeded that of the general medical practitioners.

Within the hierarchy of the British Medical Association, it has tradition-ally been general practitioners who held most of the senior positions and chaired the most important committees. This is partly due to the democratic structure of the BMA and the fact that general practitioners form the largest voting constituency. Yet it has always been the consultants in the BMA and outside it who have commanded the greater political influence at national level.

It is not easy to explain these paradoxes but they are matters of concern to general practice when power structures and society values fail to reflect their contribution to the service overall. It is often said that it has proved difficult for health authorities and public health doctors to engage with general practitioners because of their independent practitioner status. The implication is that it is easy to deal with consultants because of their employee status; in fact, almost 50 years of employment have done little to weaken the hold on freedom which hospital consultants have always enjoyed. Consequently, the self-employment of general practitioners is probably not responsible for different attitudes by the authorities. Underpinning all relationships with the medical profession is its jealously protected and continuing independence; the familiarity with consultants and specialists which district health authorities have long had contrasts with the more distant relationship with primary care. As DHAs (and their predecessor area health authorities and hospital management committees) held most of the resources and made most of the decisions about health service structures, their distance from general practice explains to some extent the relative weakness of the influence of primary care.

The fundholding scheme and its extension into total purchasing has blown this history to shreds. While consultants and specialists reside in NHS trusts, health authorities and general practitioners are moving closer together in strategies to improve health care. These new partnerships between DHAs and primary care, and their union in attempting to alter the services provided by trusts, changes the balance of power within medicine. The 1991 reforms commenced a period in which government became more dependent on general practice for the fulfilment of its goals and general practice was not found wanting.

It is possible, of course, that political change will reverse some of the structural changes of the early 1990s, especially fundholding, but it seems very unlikely that general practitioners will be deprived of the influence they now have. One day, we expect, a political adviser will have the brilliant idea of combining all the elements of the NHS in a given geographical area (health authorities, general practice and the hospital and community services) and managing them in a single entity!

The extension of partnership

Much has been said and written about the transfer of clinical responsibility from hospital to primary care, usually in debates about the failure to transfer resources accordingly. Yet despite these often unwanted shifts in the location of care, general practice remains much the same in its basic structure and culture. Surely if the nature of the work in primary care has changed so much then the skills available to deal with it should change too.

Much of the significant growth in primary care staffing in recent years has been in the form of part-time women partners in the practice and the employment of additional nursing staff, and to a lesser extent, others such as physiotherapists and counsellors. At the same time, GP referrals to hospital out-patient clinics continue to rise, albeit less quickly in fundholders, and hospital admissions are rising faster than ever. Perhaps the future shape of primary care practice combines these observations with the extension of the practice to include specialists. Most child health, elderly medicine and mental health is now conducted outside hospital – why not within the practice? And can NHS trusts learn to relate to extended general practice with their own business being transferred to primary care? Of particular note is the future place of community nursing and related services in relation to general practice. The management of these services by trusts is an accident of history rather than design and their logical home is alongside all other primary care services. The potential transfer of these staff to general practices is now enhanced by the admission of practice staff to the NHS pension scheme from September 1997.

There is also a debate to be held about the basic structure of practices in primary care. Although there are an increasing number of large practices, say ten or more partners, and a reduction in single-handed practitioners which the most recent reform proposals will accelerate, the basic unit of general practice remains the two or three-partner practice. This unit does not provide a suitable basis for extension of the primary care team, the development of specialization within the practice nor the skill framework for evidence-based medicine and for the development of the secondary care commissioning role. The creation of larger and more flexible practices is generally desirable for all of these as well as increasing the cost-effectiveness of the management arrangements for primary care. However, some patients do prefer the small practice model with the continuity and personal relationship which it offers, and some practitioners prefer it for the same reasons.

The power thing again

In many ways it was surprising that the NHS reforms were necessary to expose the potential power of primary care over specialist colleagues. More than half of all consultants and specialists rely substantially on private practice to support their lifestyles. Almost all surgeons, anaesthetists, gynaecologists and radiologists secure a high proportion of their income from private practice and the vast majority of private referrals are initiated by general practitioners. So why did they not exercise this power before?

The probability is that power broking has never been part of the culture of primary care and that exercising influence was too difficult given the distance of DHAs from the reality of primary care. The NHS reforms, and fundholding in particular, created a new culture and set of relationships between primary care and hospitals which is now being interpreted as a power struggle. In fact it may be more altruistic than that: general practitioners may genuinely have the needs of their practice population in mind as these relationships develop; after all, for many practitioners, the practice is a lifelong investment.

Party politics and primary care

At the present time, the British electorate appear to be presented with a choice of two conservative parties. Traditionally, and presumably to be restored eventually, the Conservative party favours the independence of general practice as an example of small business, and seeks to promote a mixed economy of private and public sector provision in health care. The Labour party has had a yearning for a salaried service in primary care with potentially the direction of labour in pursuit of greater equality of access to health services. Labour has always been the champion of public sector provision although its current stance is more social democratic in nature, recognizing the inevitability of the mixed economy, and the removal of current freedoms and prospective choices seems improbable.

If we have another long spell of Conservative government, it is likely that the recent moves towards privatization in one form or another will be further developed. The financial regime of NHS trusts is similar to that used by the public utilities such as water, electricity and British Telecom immediately prior to their privatization, and it is quite possible that the assets owned by NHS trusts, estimated at over £20 billion, could be sold to the private sector. The purchasing arrangements for health care would be further devolved to primary care-based total purchasing schemes with, effectively, the privatization of NHS purchasing.

In the event of a long spell of Labour government, a gradual return to traditional values is likely as political and public confidence grows. It is difficult to see how general practitioners can be excluded from debates which have become their ground during the 1990s. The growing benefits of the partnership between health authorities and general practitioners will not be discarded by a change of political colour. However, the fundholding scheme in its present form is unlikely to endure because of the ability to spend surpluses from the fund on premises owned by the practice and also due to the exposition of the unequal nature of practices respectively in, and out, of the scheme. Other characteristics of the reforms, such as clinical audit, research and development and prescribing controls, are almost certain to continue and, very probably, be further strengthened.

References

1 Department of Health, Welsh Office (1996) *Statement of Fees and Allowances Payable to General Medical Practitioners in England and Wales.*
2 HMSO (1996) Statutory Instruments 709 and 710 National Health Service, England and Wales (The Health Authorities Act 1995).
3 Department of Health (1988) *Promoting Better Health.* HMSO, London.
4 Department of Health (1989) *Working for Patients.* HMSO, London.
5 Department of Health (1989) *Practice Budgets for General Medical Practitioners* (working paper 3). HMSO, London.
6 Audit Commission (1996) *What the Doctor Ordered: A Study of GP Fundholders in England and Wales.* HMSO, London.
7 Audit Commission (1996) *Fundholding Facts. A Digest of Information about Practices within the Scheme During the First Five Years.* HMSO, London.
8 Wilson RPH (1995) Alterations in prescribing by general practitioner fundholders: an observational study. *BMJ.* **311**:1347–50.
9 NHS Executive (1994) *Developing NHS Purchasing and GP Fundholding: Towards a Primary Care-Led NHS* (EL(94)79). NHSE, Leeds.
10 Department of Health (1996) *Choice and Opportunity.* HMSO, London.
11 Department of Health (1992) *The Health of the Nation.* HMSO, London.

3

Evidence-based medicine in general practice

It is clearly the duty of the doctor to use the most economic and efficacious treatment available.[1]

Evidence-based medicine builds upon, rather than disparages or neglects, the evidence gained from good clinical skills and sound clinical experience. It is the resulting systematic search for, and incorporation of, the valid and useful subset of this evidence that keeps clinicians up to date and effective.[2]

The NHS R&D strategy and beyond

Professor Michael Peckham was appointed the first NHS Director of Research and Development in 1990. He introduced his proposals for a strategic approach to R&D for the NHS in a speech at the Royal College of Physicians, stating that:

A research approach has not been brought to bear systematically on issues relating to the effectiveness of clinical practice, the dispersal and use of existing knowledge, the best use of human and other resources, and the contributions of medical interventions to the health status of individuals and the population. Neither has there been a systematic attempt to relate important health issues to the national effort in medical research ... The challenge now is to introduce a sensible mechanism for handling within the NHS the output of basic and applied research and to apply research methods to examine the content and delivery of health care. Such a mechanism is the only way of resisting the sometimes unreasonable and often unproven resource-consuming demands of lay, professional and industrial pressure groups.[3]

Thus was the NHS R&D strategy born, with three clear major objectives: to make NHS decision-making research based; to provide the NHS with the capacity to identify problems appropriate to research; and to improve the relationship of the NHS with the science base as a whole, rather than solely with medical research.[4] Whilst the strategy was justifiably remarkable in many ways, it is also noteworthy that it made no reference to primary care and contained no focus on the first contact which characterizes the overwhelming majority of health care transactions within the NHS.

The initial phases of the 'Peckham revolution' can be seen as addressed to the funders, managers and 'doers' of R&D, albeit with a clear acknowledgement of the centrality of effectively disseminating the products of research. Furthermore, to be fair to the architects of the strategy, it must be said that there was, and is, an explicit recognition that however effective, dissemination is not synonymous with implementation. Nevertheless, one cannot but be suspicious that it has been an industrial strategy which chose to minimize the reality of its service delivery end. In part, this was a product of the overarching intent of the strategy, an intention to start before the clinical application of knowledge by dealing with the very construction of knowledge. It also reflected the domination of the financial elements of the R&D equation, in particular, questions about the costs of higher added value care reflected in the fact that health technology assessment was provided with the only standing group and permanent programme amongst the initial list of priorities. However, even whilst attention began to focus on the services provided by the staff within NHS trusts, in other words, in the major and obvious cost centres of the industry, primary care was, by and large, nowhere to be seen. In such a context, the relative weakness of the primary care research framework in the UK offered little in terms of providing a voice for primary care concerns. How was the constituency to be addressed when only one of the 1991 27-strong Central Research and Development Committee was 'out' as being from a primary care background (incidentally, a professor of general practice, listed as having interests in deprivation, health promotion, respiratory infections and terminal care). Similarly, only one of the first wave of regional R&D directors has come from a primary care background.

The NHS R&D strategy was and is, above all, an industrial strategy intended to enable the service to change its R&D behaviour from the health equivalent of the then failing IBM into something looking rather more like Bill Gates' Microsoft. At the same time that this approach was being unveiled, the doors of the 'industry' itself were being thrown open to the possibility of unprecedented and unpredictable change – the notion of a primary care-led NHS, something with altogether more anarchic potential.

The advent of the R&D strategy has prompted consideration of the relationship between a number of hitherto diverse and previously apparently hermetically sealed elements of NHS endeavour and activity, namely: research and development; clinical audit; clinical effectiveness (in terms of proven effectiveness) and the consequent notion of evidence-based medicine (EBM) or 'knowing what there is to know'. To this heady brew, discussions and debates on cost-effectiveness and 'rationing' have been added, fuelling passions regarding the clinical autonomy of doctors (the claim to self-management and consequent rejection of external controls), particularly in relation to general practice. Intimately intertwined with the question of autonomy are the questions raised in any discussion of the implementation of 'evidence' in a clinical setting, namely, the cry that 'life's not like that', manifested in complaints about 'cookbook' medicine (Box 3.1).[5]

Box 3.1: 'Cookbook' medicine – a cautionary tale[5]

'The first effective example of organized medicine is to be found in Egypt where the father figure of medicine practised – Imhotep, who was the archetypal combination of physician, priest and court official. The papyri discovered in the nineteenth century indicate that Egyptian medicine was comparatively advanced as early as the second millennium BC. Several features of that organization are outstanding in their relation to modern practice ... Rather rigid rules were laid down as to experimental treatment – there was no culpability in failure to cure so long as the standard textbooks were followed. Severe penalties were, however, threatened for those who ignored the instructions, the reason being that very few men would be expected to know better than the best specialists who had gone before'. Similarly, the Babylonian Code of Hammurabi (c.1900 BC) 'tabled penalties for negligent failure, some of which were draconian to an extent that must have deterred many from entering the profession'.

In contrast, a recent survey 'provides evidence that considerable effort is being put into creating explicit standards of care at the primary–secondary interface, but there is little evidence that these are effective' and whilst the NHS R&D programme has identified the interface as one of its priorities, with guidelines as a key area, 'it is a matter of urgency that methods are found to link the enthusiasm of local producers of guidelines with the resources and expertise of national bodies such as the Royal Colleges and specialist societies'.[6] Such activities, whilst laudable, are as likely to be focused on the creation of effective consensus as they are on the stimulation of evidence-based practice (still less the development of clinical effectiveness). Despite this downbeat (though no less accurate for it) conclusion, we do know something about how to get professionals to both 'do the right thing' and to 'do it right' (see Box 3.2).[7]

Box 3.2: Getting the right things done right[7]

Five preconditions for an ideal world:

- full specification of the appropriate technology (defined as the drugs, devices and medical and surgical procedures used in medical care, and the organizational and supportive systems within which such care is provided) must be known (or known about and easily available) to health professionals likely to encounter relevant patients

- the required combination of resources (drugs, equipment, facilities, skills and time) must be available for each relevant technology

- the number of links in the chain of practitioner action must be minimal

- professionals must be motivated to use the appropriate technology

- there must be no disincentives for professionals to utilize the appropriate technology.

We also know that:

- what is appropriate is often not fully specified (e.g. consensus conferences produce lowest common denominator compromise or employ vague language)

- specific educational interventions centring on guidelines are the most single effective method of communication

- communications are more influential when targeted on the specific practitioner (e.g. by an educationally influential preceptor or by a local product champion) and that combinations of education and data feedback are better than single approaches

- fast feedback on own behaviour enhances compliance.

In an exploration of the issues surrounding our inability to practise what is preached, Harrison has observed that we require an organizational culture in which learning, for both clinicians and policy makers, is facilitated. His survey suggests that this would be a different learning model from that implied by a 'top-down' approach (learning by following guidelines), or a 'bottom-up' approach (that learning is, in effect, random). In surveying recent evidence he concluded that 'clinical doctors do not think about the effectiveness of interventions in the same way as do epidemiologists and health service researchers, that is, in terms of "certainty about probability". Rather, such clinicians are more influenced by their own past experiences with their own patients and by the experiences of their close colleagues or mentors'. This, he suggests, can be seen as a perspective on the difference between efficacy and effectiveness.[8] By implication, his conclusions say much for the likely success of the 'top-down' approach implied in a centrally led R&D strategy.

In organizational terms, the answer perhaps rests not on an obsession with implementation failures, but more with a clustering of key features, namely the R&D process, truly clinical (rather than solely medical) audit, and clinical effectiveness, manifested as evidence-based medicine.

It's not as bad as it seems

The issues are the same for hospital specialist and GP alike – the same aspirations are required, as are the outcomes (see Box 3.3,[9] where the authors could be accused of self-justification, if not quite self-congratulation). Whilst this may be more feasible in the larger practice where a greater number of partners are able to provide a greater degree of 'specialization'

Box 3.3: Inpatient general medicine is evidence based[9]

'For many years clinicians have had to cope with the accusation that only 10–20% of the treatments they provide have any scientific foundation. Their interventions, in other words, are seldom "evidence based". Is the profession guilty as charged?

In April 1995, a general medical team at a university-affiliated district hospital in Oxford, UK, studied the treatments given to all 109 patients managed during that month on whom a diagnosis had been reached. Medical sources (including databases) were then searched for randomized controlled trial (RCT) evidence that the treatments were effective. The 109 primary treatments were then classified: 82% were evidence based (i.e. there was RCT support [53%] or unanimity on the team about the existence of convincing non-experimental evidence [29%]).

This study, which needs to be repeated in other clinical settings and for other disciplines, suggests that earlier pessimism over the extent to which evidence-based medicine is already practised is misplaced.'

in the main areas of both 'referred-on' and 'retained' patients, we should also recognize that we have been referring to the 'medical'. In a more broadly 'clinical' definition, all members and potential members of the primary health care team can act in such a way as to minimize the effect of having fewer doctors (relative to the 'demands' of patients and additional tasks described above, rather than fewer doctors in any absolute sense). The key issue, surely, is not to mimic hospital practice of an often ill-defined 'interest'. Rather, it is to reflect the aspiration for the secondary care specialist/sub-specialist of the future, whilst retaining the holistic power and perspective of general practice. In other words, what is required is the generalist who understands the limits of medical generalism, while at the same time sustaining the potency of such generalist medical input into the patient's social milieu.

Similarly, few GPs need to be told of the complications inherent in the distinction between general medical practice and the delivery of primary care services, apparent in the obvious dichotomy between the GP's practice list and the trust's locality management structure (and, for that matter, the health authority's statutory obligations towards the entire population of the health district). Who is in charge? And of what, exactly? Nor do GPs need reminding of the tension inherent in the relationship between, for example, community nursing with its history of professional practice un-managed by doctors in general, and general medical practice (indeed, some elements of community nursing are explicit in their rejection of 'medicalization'). The challenge is, undoubtedly, to deliver primary care through a team of complementary skills, rather than general medical practice with other professions subordinated. No professional group should be able to hide behind notions of professional autonomy as the only justification for any form of professional practice. The only available justification for professional practice should be that it is explicitly clinically and cost-effective. In other words, evidence based and audited.

In fact, it's quite promising

To develop an understanding of how to translate the precepts identified above, we can look to two quite different examples. The first is a systematic project-based approach – the Framework for Appropriate Care Throughout Sheffield (FACTS) – whilst the second relates the experience of a suburban teaching general practice in Leeds. The FACTS project was stimulated by the acknowledgement that the perceived independence and idiosyncrasy of GPs implies that managing changes in their behaviour presents the greatest challenge in a health care world full of challenging professional behaviours. The project team have listed the criteria for any programme of change in general practice, and have identified the techniques which help promote change (see Box 3.4). Three key facts have emerged. First, changes are more likely if making them makes life easier; secondly, flexibility, in the form of practice-based adaptation of evidence, is essential; thirdly, there is a clear need for mutual understanding between the different NHS cultures. The message for managers, particularly health authority managers, is the

---

Box 3.4: FACTS of life[10]

Choosing a programme area for change in general practice:

- Is there good evidence for changing practice?

- Is the proposed change clearly defined?

- Can the likely barriers be overcome, at least in theory?

- Is the issue relevant locally?

- Is the issue common enough to warrant the effort?

- Are significant health service resources involved?

- Can the effects of change be monitored?

- Will the programme enhance collaboration between general practices?

Techniques to help promote change:

- synthesized evidence

- endorsement by local and respected consultants

- promotional materials for recruiting practices and prompting clinicians

- practice-based, PGEA-approved training programmes

- a 'ready-made' audit programme

- administrative aids such as identifying stickers for casenotes

- individualized advice and guidance for practices

- patient leaflets and letters for use by GPs

need to 'adopt a "customer-centred" attitude – the customers being the GPs and practice staff' having previously taken the 'time and energy to understand the culture, pressures and possibilities of general practice'.[10] A rather different approach to understanding and checking behaviour (though similar in style to the hospital department study in Box 3.3) has been recorded in a retrospective analysis of consecutive consultations over two days in one practice. The authors reported that 'for each consultation, two of the authors independently recorded the primary diagnosis and intervention before reaching consensus. The primary diagnosis was defined as the first problem recorded for the consultation and the primary intervention as "the treatment or manoeuvre that represented the practitioner's attempt to cure, alleviate or care for the patient in respect of the primary diagnosis". The evidence for the interventions was then searched for in Medline (1966–95), standard textbooks and pharmaceutical companies' databases'. The authors thus described an 81% evidence-based practice (at least in terms of a combination of proven effectiveness, guidelines and consensus). They also identified two areas requiring further work: 'that standard definitions of diagnosis and interventions in general practice are unclear'; and that 'evidence derived from different methodologies may be important for the assessment of the evidence base of general practice'.[11]

EBM in general practice is not impossible and it does not mean surrendering autonomy, or credibility in the eyes of patients. In more 'structural' terms, those of accountability, it will not be long before GPs will be required to respond to the increasingly obligatory question (because of both NHS Executive sponsorship and individual and collective patient articulation), 'but will it work Doctor?'[12] However, a small-scale survey of GPs published in 1995 suggested, at least in the context of 'demanding' and/or 'articulate' patients 'that many GPs still prefer a relationship with their patients that is asymmetrical rather than symmetrical in structure, in which doctors control how it is organized'.[13] Increasingly, however, this asymmetry is being challenged – and not just by those in 'doctor-bashing' mode, but rather by those on the 'same side', whose concerns are not dissimilar to those of doctors. Both doctor and patient increasingly share a concern that the clinical and cost-effective imperatives of EBM need to be carefully balanced, so that medical decision-making is properly informed both by clinical experience (in this setting, the holistic provision of care) and by the preferences of patients. In addition, the GP also carries the weight of the patients' expectations that the other providers of primary, community, secondary and tertiary care to which they may be referred, is equally appropriately scientific. In short, all care given can and should be evidence based, even if this is only to the extent of acknowledging that there is no evidence that it is inconclusive (see Box 3.5[14]). For it to be truly effective, however, both doctor and patient need to acknowledge and respect each other's autonomy in its implementation.

Box 3.5: Dawes' four solutions[14]

- Evidence for more than a tiny fraction of the decisions made in primary care cannot possibly be available.

    'Ten years ago this may have been a legitimate argument, but today it is no longer the case ... A lot of high quality, relevant evidence is already there, but it remains invisible to most GPs, even those who keep up to date with the mainstream journals.'

- Even if the evidence were available, family practitioners could not find the time to track it down.

    'Of course they could not. But the move toward a more evidence-based primary health care does not require that practitioners track down evidence on every question or appraise all the evidence themselves. Much of the evidence that answers clinical questions in primary care has already been tracked down, critically appraised, and packaged in easily accessible forms ... The practitioner who can find one hour a week in which to search and read will make huge strides.'

- Family practitioners lack the skills and experience to critically appraise the evidence and determine its applicability within their locality.

    'Courses and workshops in critical appraisal ... are now also being run in the United Kingdom ... and increasing numbers of undergraduate and postgraduate courses are teaching these skills.'

- The relevant evidence cannot be recalled during the consultation when the answers are required.

    'With computers on the desks of a growing number of practitioners, pre-appraised evidence ... and reference-managing software, the potential exists for keeping the evidence needed to assist with the most frequent questions and decisions literally at one's fingertips.'

Off-the-shelf information and experience

The starting point for anyone seeking relevant, high quality information in the NHS is the ability to arrange the words 'wheat' and 'chaff' into a well-known phrase or saying. In a world of 10 000 journals, on what basis should the aspiring practitioner start to search? In attempting to answer the question 'what clinical information do doctors need?', the editor of the *British Medical Journal* has recently reviewed the management of clinical information[14] and attempted to provide a hierarchy of usefulness which can be adapted to the quest for information on the appropriate and proven clinically effective care, its organization and commissioning.

In summarizing his review of information needs, Smith makes three salient points: that doctors use some two million pieces of information to manage patients; that textbooks, journals and other existing information tools are not adequate; and that the best information sources provide relevant, valid material that can be accessed quickly and with minimal effort. Combining Smith's view of the information needs of individual doctors managing individual patients and Dawes' positive approach (see Box 3.5) to evidence-based medicine, offers the possibility of a simple 'beginner's guide' to the most readily available (and often most heavily touted) sources.

At the top of Smith's hierarchy come four information sources: evidence-based, regularly updated textbooks; systematic journal reviews; portable summary of systematic reviews; and the Internet in 10 years' time. Each of these is judged to have high relevance, validity and usefulness while requiring low work to access them. The second tier (moderate to high relevance, validity and usefulness, still only requiring low work) includes: drug reference books; the current forerunners of systematic abstract journals; and colleagues. The third category (mainly low to moderate in terms of relevance, validity and usefulness with uniformly moderate work required) embraces standard textbooks and journal reviews; collections of systematic reviews; consensus statements, clinical guidelines and on-line searching. The least powerful category includes journal articles and the Internet as it currently stands.

Given that the most powerful sources are a description of potential, our classification outlines elements in a more modest reality.

The future will look like this

- *ACP Journal Club on Disk* (serial software for PC or Macintosh). Haynes RB, editor, American College of Physicians, Philadelphia

- *Evidence-Based Medicine* (BMJ Publishing, tel. 0171 383 6185)

And these are worth more than a passing glance

- *UK Cochrane Centre* (produces systematic, up-to-date reviews of randomized controlled trials of health care interventions). Available on disk and CD-ROM as The Cochrane Library, comprising: the database of systematic reviews; the database of abstracts of reviews of effectiveness; the controlled trials register; the database of reviews methodology. From BMJ Publishing, PO Box 295, London WC1H 9TE. Tel. 0171 383 6185; UK Cochrane Centre, Summertown Pavilion, Middle Way, Oxford OX2 7LG, Website http://hiru.mcmaster.ca/COCHRANE/DEFAULT.HTM

- *CRD* (NHS Centre for Reviews and Dissemination for Effectiveness Matters; *Effective Health Care* bulletins; database of abstracts of reviews of effectiveness (DARE); Cochrane databases, including database of systematic reviews). University of York, York YO1 5DD. Fax. 01904 433661; e-mail: revdis@york.ac.uk or the Web to http://www.york.ac.uk/inst/crd/welcome.htm. DARE is available on the Internet (Telnet to nhscrd.york.ac.uk, with the username crduser and password crduser) and as part of the Cochrane Library

- *Bandolier* (monthly newsletter on evidence-based health care), c/o Pain Research, The Churchill, Oxford OX3 7LJ. Fax. 01865 226978; e-mail: andrew.moore%mailgate@jr2.ox.ac.uk. Accessible on the Web at http://www.jr2.ox.ac.uk/Bandolier

- *Evidence-Based Purchasing* (bi-monthly selection of new material) available from: Information and Communications Coordinator, R&D Directorate, Canynge Hall, Whiteladies Road, Bristol BS8 2PR

- *Medical libraries* (for example, self- or librarian-assisted Medline searching; plus access to the Internet)

- *Royal Colleges*

- *FACTS* (Framework for Appropriate Care Throughout Sheffield), c/o Medical Care Research Unit, University of Sheffield, Sheffield

- *PACE* (Promoting Action on Clinical Effectiveness) – 16 local implementation projects – contact: King's Fund Development Centre, 11–13 Cavendish Square, London W1M 0AN

- *Centre for Primary Care Research,* University of Manchester, Oxford Road, Manchester M13 9PL

- *Health authorities and NHS Executive regional offices* (R&D Information Manager or equivalent and Clinical Audit Coordinator or equivalent) for details of local programmes and initiatives; national programmes; access to the NHS research register (register of research taking place in the NHS)

- *University departments of general practice*

References

1 British Medical Association (1984) *Handbook of Medical Ethics*, p. 67. BMA, London.
2 Sackett D L (1995) Evidence-based medicine. *Lancet.* **346**:840.
3 Peckham M (1991) Research and development in the National Health Service. *Lancet* **338**:367–71.
4 Peckham M (1991) *Research for Health.* Department of Health, London.
5 Mason J K and McCall Smith R A (1983) *Law and Medical Ethics*, pp. 4–5. Butterworths, London.
6 Littlejohns P and Sharda A (1995) Guidelines and protocols for sharing of health care between hospitals and general practitioners. *Medical Audit News.* **5**(2):24–5.
7 Harrison S (1994) Knowledge into practice: what's the problem? *Translating Knowledge into Practice* (Regional R&D Task Force Report), pp. 11–13. Yorkshire Regional Health Authority, Harrogate.
8 Harrison S (1995) Implementing the results of research in clinical and managerial practice. In M Baker and S Kirk (eds) *Research and Development for the NHS*, p. 111. Radcliffe Medical Press, Oxford.
9 Ellis J, Mulligan I, Rowe J *et al.* (1995) Inpatient general medicine is evidence based. *Lancet.* **346**:407–10.
10 Munro J (1995) Facing the FACTS. *Health Service Journal*, 5 October: 26–7.

11 Gill P, Dowell A C, Neal R D *et al.* (1996) Evidence-based general practice: a retrospective study of interventions in one training practice. *BMJ.* **312**:819–21.

12 See, for example, King's Fund Consumer Health Information Project; Promoting Patient Choice; Midwives Information & Resource Service; Help for Health Trust; featured in (1996) *King's Fund News.* **19**:1.

13 Calnan M and Williams S (1994) Challenges to professional autonomy in the United Kingdom? The perceptions of general practitioners. *International Journal of Health Services.* **25**(2):219–41.

14 Smith R (1996) What clinical information do doctors need? *BMJ.* **313**: 1062–8.

4

A hierarchy of primary care needs

Primary care is the nearest experience to reality which the health industry offers. The pressures of service delivery are set close by the tensions of modern private living. We recently asked a friend who is a general practitioner to list the immediate problems he faced. He came up with this list:

'*Practice*

- Partner off sick last three months.

- Is making good recovery but is retiring on grounds of ill health.

- Locums difficult to find in the short term.

- Will the health authority and the Local Medical Committee support our application and will the Medical Practices Committee approve a full-time replacement GP – our list is small and has fallen slightly in the last two years.

- Will we be able to find a replacement GP?

- Small list size, low earning practice, above average expenses. Quiet part of the country – perhaps a long way from family and existing friends of incoming partner.

- Senior receptionist told me today her husband's job has been moved to the Midlands and she has given two weeks' notice.

- Will need to recruit new senior receptionist or promote one of the existing receptionists and then recruit her replacement. Either course of action is potentially disruptive and training will need to be funded and arranged.

- In the short term, someone who knows what they are doing needed to cover SR's hours. Where can I find someone in two weeks?

- Practice computer system and patient notes are in a mess.

- Most of the partners would like to use the practice computer instead of paper records now. We all keep some written records and some on the computer so there is no complete record in either system. As well as being frustrating in the clinical situation we are worried about making a serious clinical mistake with medico-legal consequences. One partner dislikes using the computer when consulting with patients and so far we have not been able to persuade her of the benefits.

Finances

- Need to do a stocktake.

- Retiring partner will need share of premises and contents (capital and current accounts); incoming partner needs to be able to purchase – loan to arrange.

- Practice accounts for previous year not yet available from accountant.

- Practice manager currently off sick and due to retire in nine months.

- Bookkeeping currently in a mess. I am doing the basics as best I can (at least the staff get their pay cheques on time) but it is a task for which I have received no training.

- When accountant's queries on last year's books come in who is there to provide the answers?

- Will need to recruit replacement – what is the quality of person available for the scale of pay we can offer? Can I persuade the health authority to increase the practice staff budget?

- Will need to look at job description – retiring partner used to perform some functions that I think could be done by the practice manager.

Domestic/family

- Wife is expecting baby in five months. She is well and we are both very happy at the prospect. But we need the builders who are putting in a new central heating system and replacing the leaking roof to get a move on so we can get the decorating finished before the baby arrives.

Personal

- I would like to take my oldest son to the football more often, my wife to the theatre more often, have a weekend walking in the Lakes with some old university friends next month. How do I find the time?

Professional

- The other local practices in our out-of-hours cooperative want to make changes – persuade more patients to come to us rather than us do home visits and extend the hours the co-op works. We are already doing our sick partner's share of the work and we cannot contemplate more changes at the moment.

Audit

- We are committed to reviewing a sample of patient notes of those who have hypertension and to looking at our standards of care. The deadline for the initial review and return to the Medical Audit Advisory Group (MAAG) coordinator was last week but the partner involved is on holiday. We had a reminder phone call from the MAAG today. I think we are holding up the project.

Local commissioning

- The health authority and other local practices want us to get involved. I don't know what it means never mind whether I want to get involved.

Clinical problems

- I saw 186 people last week. I've a 49-year-old woman dying of ovarian cancer, a chap I saw last night with severe headaches that might be something serious but probably isn't and a baby I saw earlier today with a temperature that I need to re-examine on the way home. There are three or four of my elderly regulars who could really do with assessment by a social worker but the offices are always engaged when I try and ring them. The Community Psychiatric Nurse (CPN) thinks one of my young schizophrenics is relapsing. The midwife thinks one of my antenatal patients is small for dates. I don't, but is the midwife a more expert clinician in her field than me?

Do you want me to go on?'

The practice, the problems and the timescale are genuine. The issues, though not usually so concentrated in time and place, are widely reflected and understood in NHS general practice.

Clinical effectiveness is not at the top of our friend's list of problems to be addressed, but he is aware of it as an issue. How can he be helped? Not surprisingly he finds it difficult to comprehend how he can deliver care to his patients that he knows to be the right thing in the right way at the right time on every occasion. He is busy 'fire-fighting' on both the practice management front and the clinical front. Quite rightly he thinks he is doing a good job under difficult circumstances. But our friend remains uneasy. He is worried about the lack of facilities for single parents, many of whom live in poor housing, and thinks a children's day centre could do more good for the health of children and parents than he can. He is concerned at the local trust spending £250 000 setting up a new laboratory to do cardiac catheterizations when the hospital ten miles away offers a perfectly satisfactory service. Will this improve the health of the population or just develop health care? He knows that any audit he has done shows room for improvement in the care he and his partners are providing. He knows that the overspend on the practice drug budget could be turned into an underspend with clear practice policies and a concerted effort from all partners. Above all, he knows that change and challenges have been a feature of general practice and primary care since the creation of the National Health Service in 1948.

Health authorities, academics and others promoting clinical effectiveness in primary care need to be aware of the problems of general practitioners, what the basic requirements are for a practice to move from fire-fighting into the planning and management mode required to change clinical practice, and to understand how to facilitate that process. General practitioners also need to understand the causes and potential solutions to some of their current difficulties and to be prepared to meet these new challenges with the same innovation and cooperation that has characterized UK general practice from at least the mid-1960s. This chapter addresses these issues.

The grief reaction

The 1966 GP charter created subsidies for group practices, larger and better equipped premises, and the employment of other primary care staff. The payments from the State for general medical services (GMS) involved approximately 50% of practice income being generated by a fixed basic practice allowance plus capitation payments increasingly weighted by age, and 50% from item of service payments, e.g. cervical cytology and immunization of children. The former could be regarded as basic pay and the latter as performance-related pay. The 1966 changes were regarded as progressive and with relief by general practitioners.

The NHS reforms of 1989 and 1990 created fundholding and continued with the GMS subsidies from 1966. The State payments were only marginally adjusted in cash terms with 55% 'basic pay' and 45% 'perform-ance related'. However, a reduced basic practice allowance and increased capitation payments, together with all-or-nothing target payments for cer-vical cytology and immunizations, changed the culture of primary care – particularly when the following years have seen restricted funds for further developments funded from the traditional routes. Limited subsidies con-tinue to be available for the development of information technology (with larger amounts going to fundholding practices), but additional cash for premises and staff has been severely restrained following a burst of growth in numbers (particularly practice nurses) around the time of the reforms. The changes were generally regarded with despair and anger by GPs – increased work, power and responsibility as fundholders for an increasing number was accompanied by uncertainty about the future and perceived financial insecurity – feelings which have not been dispelled by the passage of time.

Several years on, whilst the initial grief reaction for 'general practice as we knew it' has subsided, increasing workload (both in primary care and shifted from secondary care), an increasingly informed and/or demanding public, continuing technical and pharmacological advances, concern about recruitment of locums and partners and universal exhortations to develop the 'primary care-led NHS' are standard fare. There is the paradigm ex-ploding out of the 1995 out-of-hours arrangements whereby many more general practitioners have delegated the out-of-hours care of their patients to others, a response to a genuine problem with potentially far-reaching consequences. The accountability framework for purchasing (including the development of total purchasing projects), together with the continuing re-accreditation debate, creates uncertainty over future accountability for primary care provision.

Lists similar to our friend's could be generated by many UK general practitioners. Are GPs adaptable enough to accommodate continuing shifts in their expected roles and ways of working?

The pace of change

This pace of change is not confined to UK general practice or even to medi-cine. The loss of practice stability mirrors the reconstruction of employment options across the economy. Tom Peters wrote *Thriving on Chaos*[1] at the end of the 1980s, and 10 years on the privatized British Telecom makes billions of pounds of profit annually yet at the same time has shed 20 000 jobs in the last two years. The newly privatized power industries are following the same path. International currencies used to fluctuate less than 1% a year, now 10% in turbulent years is not uncommon – this revolution led to Britain's withdrawal from the European Exchange Rate Mechanism, the ripples from which continue to disturb relations with governments with which we will undoubtedly need to cooperate closely in order to produce elusive economic success.

Fragmentation of the workforce is widespread, with fewer employed in big companies and an explosion in the self-employed and in small, niche, specialized businesses. On a smaller scale some businesses have been replaced by the advance of technology. For example, copying and duplicating services which existed as stand-alone businesses in most medium-sized towns 15 years ago have been replaced by office and sometimes desktop photocopiers – the quality of copies is immeasurably better and availability is immediate. Photographic films used to be sent to Kodak and the prints would arrive back in about a week. Now we can go to almost any high street photographic shop and our pictures are available in an hour – with better quality results.

The successful copying service of 15 years ago has moved and diversified into supplying office services. The employees have trained in selling and servicing a range of products, learnt to handle computers and automated tills, and the really successful have been on public speaking and communication skill courses to become more confident and competent at handling customer relations. The response time to customer requests has also come down. GPs call this 'the Macdonald factor' and it exists. Keep someone more than 20 minutes in the waiting room beyond their appointment time and quite often a challenging consultation becomes an impossible one as dissonance between patient and doctor obscures progress towards identifying problems and their potential solutions.

Quality of service, flexibility in the service offered and quick response times are now part of the culture of society in the 1990s. Meeting these challenges is a requirement and not an option for the National Health Service; hankering for the golden years (if they really existed) of 1966 to 1989 has now become pointless and harmful. Solutions to these new problems need to be found, just as age–sex and morbidity registers, appointments and practice nurses were introduced to deliver the early chronic disease management systems and prevention programmes in primary care, two of the major challenges of the 1970s.

All clinicians strive to provide the best health care possible for their patients. Despite these endeavours, given the complexity and range of potential modern treatments, together with the myriad of presenting symptomatology in primary care, it is not surprising that almost any practice-based audit shows areas where the application of existing knowledge is less than optimum. The steps required to improve clinical performance are logical, simple and undoubtedly within the capability of any medical graduate. But before we deliver to our friend clinical-effectiveness evidence which he can use, he needs to understand where his problems are coming from and start to solve some of them. Even the best seeds need to be sown in fertile soil.

Management

To many clinicians the 'M' word remains anathema. As a social science it appears to have little hard evidence to support theories or action and biological scientists (including doctors) find this hard to take. In the same way physicians involved in teaching think (at least initially) that educational theory has little to offer them. Their past experience of management has usually been inactivity or obstructive administration, sometimes even obstruction of the *wants* of those with *clinical* responsibility. Point out to a general practitioner that in planning and supervising the building of a new surgery or selecting and installing a computer system he or she has been using high-level management skills and the usual responses are either disbelief or 'if that's the case then anyone can be a manager'. This is the point at which the argument can begin to be turned around – if someone else who had the same skills had been given the opportunity to manage those projects they ought to have been completed just as successfully but with the GP being released to see patients, with a supervisory role at most.

In fact most GPs and most practice managers are poor at managing the day-to-day issues.[2] Most practices do not have a strategy for development: clinical policies are occasionally discussed but operational policies for running the business are rarer; attention to detail often concentrates on financial matters involving a few pounds whilst receptionists responsible for the success or failure of the practice work without a pension or an annual appraisal and training programme.

Let us make the conservative estimate that a receptionist has 200 face-to-face and telephone consultations with patients in a working day, more than any other individual in the primary health care team. A patient is worth approximately £50 per year to the practice – about half in capitation fees and the rest in target income, items of service and non-NHS charges levied directly to the patient or paid by third parties, e.g. insurance companies.

If each patient stays registered for 10 years the receptionist is handling customers worth £100 000 to the practice in a single day.

Our friend would know what to do if someone sat a small group down for a quiet hour once or twice a month and planned how to react when a partner is unexpectedly taken ill, how the practice might go about recruiting a new partner and who could do the books if the practice manager left. If a real staff training programme had been in place a replacement senior receptionist (or even practice manager) would probably not only be identified but already be partially accredited.

Interpersonal communications require working at, in the same way as other aspects of primary care. If n is the number of people in a primary health care team, the number of lines of communication required is expressed by the formula $(n^2 - n) \div 2$. Thus with five people in a team there are 10 lines of communication. A team of 20 has 190 lines. The key clinical communication tool in UK general practice is the patient record and most practices have at least 20 people requiring access to clinical records for one reason or another.

It is increasingly difficult to see paper-based medical records in primary care meeting all of the requirements of a usable database. Already the majority of practices are linked with health authorities for the transfer of patient registration details. Item of service payments are increasingly to be carried out electronically and this has been the norm for dental practitioners in the UK for some time. Any strategy for clinical records developed today (instead of in 1911 as a result of Lloyd George's National Insurance Act) would have to exclude anything other than an electronic record. Symptoms and diagnoses would be coded in a uniform manner, as would advice, therapy and referral. Remote access to the practice clinical database, e.g. on home visits, is no longer experimental. Whilst confidentiality issues must always remain in the forefront of thinking when clinical records are considered, the problems are not insurmountable. More problematic is getting the agreement of the record users to use the electronic record at all, and then to do so consistently and accurately.

Assessing the usefulness of current GP computer records for purposes such as health needs assessment at practice level has produced a helpful picture of the current position. Any information collection system when assessed for the first time is likely to fall short of the users' requirements. A GP facing a complaint from a patient will often wish that his or her paper records were more legible and/or complete. Health authorities and trusts found major problems in the diagnostic coding of procedures, which was widely required for the first time in 1991 with the introduction of health care contracting. It is not surprising, therefore, to find that often not all members of a practice will record to the same level of coverage; there are differences in the definitions of symptoms and diagnoses by clinicians (my asthma is your chronic obstructive pulmonary disease); and differences between coding systems makes the use of aggregated or inter-practice data (even if it is of high quality at practice level) at best difficult and often impossible.

The problems with agreeing on methods and standards for records is an illustration of the problems facing practices across the management agenda. Too many practices have become extended organizations with appointment systems, clinical records and other processes poorly coordinated, too little attention paid to the relative importance of current activities (habits), inadequate definition of clinical and practice priorities and little knowledge of the standards of care being achieved. The primary health care team has grown in size but has this been reflected by a similar growth in stature and self-esteem of team members?

Practice administration or practice management?

With more than 90% of general practices having appointed a manager, how has this management vacuum developed? Part of the answer lies in the evolution and definition of the practice manager's role. Often appointed as a response by GPs to their need for a pair of hands to take care of the administration and organization, it seems that the task of most practice managers has been overwhelmingly one of sorting out problems with staff, systems and patients. However, there are sufficient reports of difficulties in delegation and 'letting go' by doctors and underperformance by overpromoted and undertrained managers to suggest that neither needs nor potential are being met. Surveys show that few managers have a focus external to the practice with an emphasis towards relationships with trusts, social services, housing, community health council, health authority and other local organizations.

There are two main obstacles to the development of the practice manager as a manager rather than an administrator. First, the doctors' view of 'their' practice and their position as employers of the practice manager limits the ability of colleagues to shift the focus from internal to external and from crisis management to strategy. Doctors need to be prepared to be trained in management themselves and then move into the role of executive directors, rather than perform badly in the role of middle manager. Second, the conventional practice management training available concentrates on training in skills rather than attitudinal and behavioural development. Practice managers need to be skilled in networking, working within a political environment, and to be able to think strategically and to manage change.

Both parties need these skills need to be developed in a different educational setting from those currently in place – good general management training is available for other health care professionals from a number of well-regarded organizations, e.g. King's Fund; Centre for Health Services Management at the University of Nottingham. Primary care has severely limited capacity for implementing complex issues such as those involved in changing clinical practice without this endowment of management skills within the practice team. Whilst many attempts have been made to bridge the primary care chasm that lies between practice administration and management, there are yet no clear processes or recognized successful providers to facilitate this development.

For the successful development of the practice manager both the above obstacles need to be tackled simultaneously. So often a practice will have the vision to recognize the need to tackle the relationship and responsibility issues, yet the connection is not made with the educational requirements that are appropriate to bring that about. Sometimes the obstacle is perhaps that funding is not forthcoming. The obverse situation also applies, with the educational agenda clear to the practice manager but his or her employers having difficulty in recognizing and overcoming the relationship and role obstruction. Practices can be poor employers and GPs poor managers.

The training agenda for practice managers is a small illustration of the need for a coordinated primary care response to the hectic change agenda. The mood is menacing, morale is poor. Tom Peters[1] identified two potential retorts to threats from change:

1 shifting of blame and of burdens; seeking protection from external drivers of change; grudgingly accepting what are perceived as inadequate pay offers; employing lower grades of staff at lower cost; threatening industrial action

or

2 continuously retraining all members of staff for increasingly complex tasks; automating routine tasks; increasing worker flexibility and creativity; diffusing responsibility for innovation; giving all members a stake in improved performance via profit-related schemes.

Lessons from recent history around the world, whether in the public or the private sector, show that the second response is the *only* successful riposte to the present pace of change. Everyone takes a greater responsibility for the soundness and efficiency of the practice. A close relationship with the external stakeholders develops and the reputation and self-esteem of the practice and those who work there soar. They, and all those associated, become partners in its future. Archie Norman and his team at Asda are a good example in the UK of what can be achieved with this approach to management – turning a supermarket retailer making big losses and ripe for take-over into an expanding and profitable company, sharing those profits with all the companies' 'colleagues' (no one just works at Asda, everyone is a colleague).

There is plenty of the first negative response around in general practice but some elements of the second are just about discernible, even if not clearly articulated. Facilitating the positive response through a rigorous management development programme at practice level needs to be a priority for practices and health authorities.

A hierarchy of needs in primary care

In order for our friend to survive his panoply of life's pressures, succeed as a primary care physician and deliver care based on clinical effectiveness, he needs to understand the hierarchy of need.

Looking closely at human motivation, a number of different ways that human behaviour responds positively or negatively to change can be identified. One of the most useful theories was first described by Abraham Maslow in 1954.[3] Maslow was a New York psychologist who rejected traditional behavioural models which were based on organisms modifying their behaviour in order to achieve a state in which they received the least stimulation possible. Many human *physiological* systems do operate in this manner and thinking at the time was heavily influenced by behaviourism based solely upon experimental evidence, usually from animals. However, Maslow recognized that a cognitive model was required since human beings often seek to optimize stimulation by their exploratory behaviour – curiosity, search for meaning and language.

He proposed that there are a number of complex needs which are interdependent and structured hierarchically (see Figure 4.1). Broadly speaking it may be considered that each different level of need is addressed when the one underneath has been satisfied. If we are in a situation where these needs are not being met then we are unable to devote time and energy to a higher level in the hierarchy until the lower level has been completed.

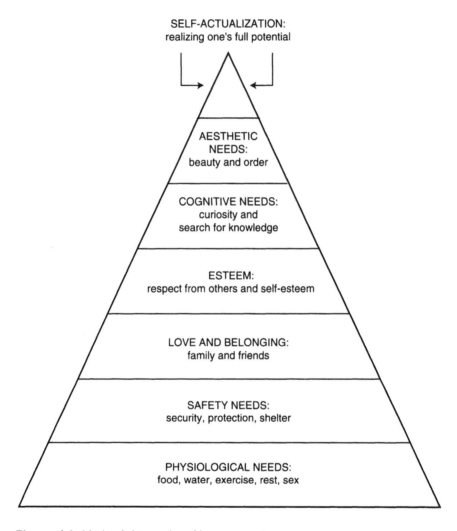

Figure 4.1 Maslow's hierarchy of human needs

Food, drink and shelter become more important than anything else if they are not available. Once secure, social needs then become the priority, and when those are no longer the driving force cognitive needs attract attention and so on.

Maslow's theory seems very useful in the work situation, mainly because it explains why workers' needs never seem to be entirely satisfied. Once adequate pay has been achieved, job satisfaction becomes the next goal. Interestingly, research shows that being overpaid as perceived by employees can be as great a source of stress and dissatisfaction as being underpaid. This supports Rogers[4] and Harre[5] who argue that the need for positive regard and social respect are the most important human motivators. It may be more important for people to be loved or approved of or respected or – at the very least – to avoid being made to look ridiculous, than anything else.

Another helpful aspect of human motivation has to do with perceived effectiveness. If dogs are exposed to unavoidable electric shocks[6] they become very passive and remain passive even in a situation where taking action would allow them to avoid further pain. This is referred to as learned helplessness[7] – the experience of being a victim can produce general apathy. Human experiments replicate the animal model. College students[8] given a series of unsolvable puzzles were later given a second series of solvable puzzles. They performed worse than students who had not had the earlier demoralizing experience.

Whilst we would acknowledge that human motivation is more complex than these simplistic models can account for, it is useful to consider the lessons that these respected theories provide in the context of primary care development.

Positive rapport and support are required for health care workers in primary care. A positive reinforcement of good practice is more likely to produce further change than only the pointing out of deficiencies. Change has left many with low self-esteem, and whilst learned helplessness may be too strong an expression of morale for some, surveys showing that 20% of general practitioners have contemplated suicide should ring warning bells amongst those with responsibilities for the health care system and for patients. Responsiveness is essential to facilitate development within primary care: people are most likely to act themselves when they feel that their own actions are having an effect, when they feel a sense of personal agency in their dealings with the world.

A hierarchy of need for primary care (Figure 4.2) can be constructed from observation. Our friend's list is an example of this since the general order of problems follows the hierarchy, with security and finance presumably the most pressing issues since they are mentioned first. Then he moves into social areas, before cognitive issues appear. Finally, self-actualization in the shape of personal growth (mixed with some social needs) completes the list. All practices at times of crisis will move into survival mode. If success is based upon esteem and respect, the most successful general practices are those which are able to spend the maximum amount of time in the areas of cognitive need and self-actualization.

Creating conditions for survival, safety, increasing self-esteem and developing cognitive skills is pretty much an essential prerequisite to primary

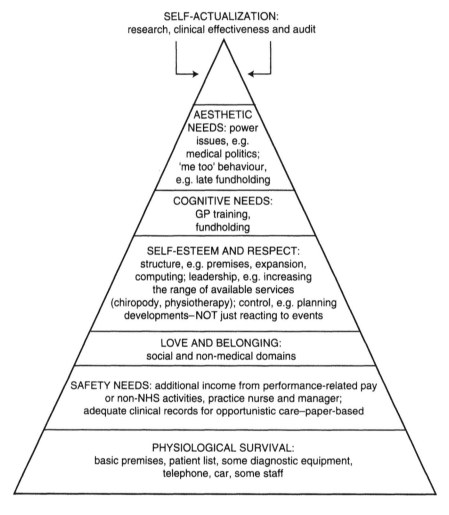

SELF-ACTUALIZATION:
research, clinical effectiveness and audit

AESTHETIC
NEEDS: power
issues, e.g.
medical politics;
'me too' behaviour,
e.g. late fundholding

COGNITIVE NEEDS:
GP training,
fundholding

SELF-ESTEEM AND RESPECT:
structure, e.g. premises, expansion,
computing; leadership, e.g. increasing
the range of available services
(chiropody, physiotherapy); control, e.g. planning
developments–NOT just reacting to events

LOVE AND BELONGING:
social and non-medical domains

SAFETY NEEDS: additional income from performance-related pay
or non-NHS activities, practice nurse and manager;
adequate clinical records for opportunistic care–paper-based

PHYSIOLOGICAL SURVIVAL:
basic premises, patient list, some diagnostic equipment,
telephone, car, some staff

Figure 4.2 A hierarchy of needs in general practice

care taking on the challenge of clinical effectiveness. These can be achieved through management yet have eluded many to date. One of the very top priorities for general practice is to put these essential building blocks in place and then deliver clinically effective health care and demonstrably improve the health of the population.

Conditions for this will not just spontaneously appear, they need to be created. Health authorities with their roles of strategy, monitoring and support are ideally placed to increasingly deliver the climate which will support these changes. Collaboration with primary health care teams, hospital trusts, local authorities, Royal Colleges, postgraduate deans, university departments and others will be required. Primary health care teams need to be aware of the strategy for primary care development, receptive to the principles involved and responsive to the challenge of this bewilderingly complex task.

References

1 Peters T (1988) *Thriving on Chaos*. Macmillan, London.
2 Rout U (1996) Occupational stress in practice managers. *Primary Care Management*. 6(1):5–9.
3 Maslow A H (1970) *Motivation and Personality* (2nd edn). Harper and Row, New York.
4 Rogers C R (1961) *On Becoming a Person: A Therapist's View of Psychotherapy*. Constable, London.
5 Harre R (1979) *Social Being*. Basil Blackwell, Oxford.
6 Seligman M E P and Maier S F (1967) Failure to escape traumatic shock. *Journal of Experimental Psychology*. 74:1–9.
7 Seligman M E P (1975) *Helplessness: On Depression, Development and Death*. W H Freeman, San Francisco.
8 de Vellis R F and Callahan L F (1993) A brief measure of helplessness. *Journal of Rheumatology*. 20:866.

5

Delivering the evidence

Today's therapy, instigated solely as a result of clinical experience, becomes tomorrow's bad joke.[1]

The concept of 'evidence-based medicine' (EBM) has received much attention in recent years. It was first advocated by Archie Cochrane in *Effectiveness and Efficiency* and has been taken on by David Sackett, now of Oxford University, and his colleagues from McMaster and Ottawa Universities.[1,2] The development of EBM is inextricably linked with the landmark publication of *Effective Care in Pregnancy and Childbirth* by Ian Chalmers and colleagues in 1989.[3] It involves the application of clinical trial evidence to everyday care as a means of closing the gap between research and everyday practice. Four steps are involved:

1 accurate identification of the question to be investigated

2 a search of the literature to select relevant articles

3 an evaluation of the evidence in the literature selected

4 implementation of the findings in clinical practice.

Given the sometimes inflated expectations that have surrounded clinical epidemiology it is not surprising that we are aware of continuing scepticism in some quarters concerning evidence-based medicine. The fears of some clinicians that these developments threaten the concept of the individual doctor–patient relationship are an understandable emotional reaction to the change threatening current practice. In fact the obverse is true. In order to deliver EBM to individual patients *greater* clinical skills are required. Diagnoses must be ever more accurate, communication skills need to be honed to a fine art to achieve a jointly agreed and understood management plan between doctor and patient, and new skills learnt to master the scientific basis of clinical practice.

It must be recognized, even by evidence-based enthusiasts, that there are limits to this approach. As knowledge about specific effective interventions becomes clearer, the difficulties of applying this knowledge and judgement to individual patients who may well have multiple pathologies or risk factors means that increased professional expertise will be demanded of doctors. As treatment improves the stakes involved in delivering optimal clinical care increase. Combining multiple interventions into clinical strategies on an evidence base is problematical. Two interventions can be combined in two different ways. Five interventions results in a possible 120 combinations. The risk of 'cookbook medicine' taking over is not credible but neither is continuing with practice based solely on opinion and clinical experience.

Continuing medical education for the 21st century

There is increasing emphasis on effectiveness and efficiency from patients and professional leaders. The challenge is to achieve the best care for individuals and the population in the face of increasing health care costs, demographic change and the pattern of disease (notably the ageing population and the increase in chronic health problems), biomedical advances and communication of knowledge previously only vested intraprofessionally. These forces lead inevitably to changing requirements in medical education.

Educational processes and learning environments need to be created in which doctors can prepare themselves for their future role. Attitudes, behaviour, flexible thinking, access to data about, and implementation of, effective care are now more important than the mere possession of biomedical information. Core knowledge of the scientific basis of medicine remains essential but training in scientific methods and in critical appraisal is becoming the driving force. Current educational activities in this area are not sufficient to support professional needs.[4] Memory becomes less important as increasingly knowledge-based computer systems provide up-to-date information. General practitioners are already familiar with drug interaction and drug-morbidity contraindication warnings on their desktops. EMIS software, one of the largest of UK suppliers, will not permit the prescribing of beta-blockers to a patient with a previous diagnosis of asthma entered onto that patient's computerized notes. This trend towards guidance systems will continue: there are already those who feel that if a patient receives inappropriate treatment for a condition which would have been warned against by a recognized electronic database in common use, then a legal case could be built against the doctor not using the available assistance.

All UK medical schools are revising their curricula following the 1993 General Medical Council recommendations[5] in line with these needs; the introduction of a critical reading paper into the postgraduate examination for membership of the Royal College of General Practitioners in 1992 is a further recognition of this change in direction. Examinations in the future will have less emphasis on memorizing long tracts of information masquerading as facts. Greater importance will be placed upon demonstrating the ability to use information to solve clinical problems and communication skills. The gauntlet has been thrown down – will those already qualified in medicine be brave enough to pick it up through their continuing education?

Can we start from here?

A visitor, lost in the byways of Ireland, stops to ask the way of a local, obviously a farmer. 'Can you tell me the way to Galway, please?' he says. The farmer scratches his head and thinks for a few seconds before he replies, 'Galway you're after? If it's Galway you're after I shouldn't be starting from here'.

Despite difficulties in progressing the elusive management developments described in Chapter 4, and therefore difficulties in finding time for cognitive and self-actualization activity, there has been real progress in beginning work towards an evidence-based health service in the UK primary care setting. Audit, in particular, has become a familiar exercise through the work of medical audit advisory groups, as well as through the chronic disease management modules for asthma and diabetes associated with the otherwise ill-designed health promotion banding arrangements.

There are some concerns that much 'audit' activity has in fact only been data collection, and therefore clinical practice and existing habits have remained unchanged. (The concerns apply perhaps even more so to 'audit' in secondary care which has been generously resourced in time and money when compared to primary care.) Despite this, we have recently found in discussions with two groups of GP registrars that basic knowledge of the key interventions based on evidence and knowledge about the ways to translate these into changed clinical practice with individual patients, is well developed.

The two groups came up with lists of interventions that were remarkably similar when asked to think about 'areas of clinical practice that they were sure were based on evidence':

- aspirin as secondary prevention in ischaemic heart disease

- streptokinase in acute myocardial infarction

- helicobacter eradication for duodenal ulceration

- beta blockade as secondary prevention post-myocardial infarction and as a reducer of cardiac events in those with hypertension

- ACE inhibitors post myocardial infarction and in heart failure

- warfarin/aspirin and atrial fibrillation

- cholesterol reduction – primary and secondary prevention of ischaemic heart disease

- combined oral contraception

- good diabetic control and tertiary prevention of vascular, renal and eye problems

- smoking cessation – primary and secondary prevention

- immunizations – Hib

- cervical cytology

- mammography

- HRT and osteoporosis

- endarterectomy for carotid stenosis.

When asked about the ways in which it could be possible to deliver these interventions to individual patients, they listed:

- clarify the question, clearly identifying the diagnosis, the appropriate patients and the intervention

- be sure that the evidence actually does support the identified topic

- set priorities in the clinically effective areas – being realistic in taking on two or three topics and doing them well

- need to obtain agreement and enthusiasm of all in PHCT to deliver change on these agreed priorities

- use practice computer systems to either set up reminders for clinicians to act upon opportunistically at the next consultation with that patient or to run a recall list of patients for specifically initiated discussions

- develop consultation skills to be able to reach an informed decision taken jointly by patient and GP

- set standards within the selected topics against which to measure the application of the effective clinical practice

- audit via the practice computer to check on whether the agreed priorities are being applied.

Whilst the groups recognized that they were less confident about their knowledge of the evidence about effectiveness in any detail, and of their ability to critically assess the wealth of literature, we received a clear demonstration of knowledge and enthusiasm on which to build. Before we consider how the evidence can be delivered to clinicians, we should ensure that the principles involved in appraising the evidence in the medical literature are familiar. Then further difficulties in delivering information can be assessed.

Chance, bias and confounding variables

In any study of the effect of a medical intervention on the natural history of a disease, one would expect to see results clearly stated. They may show that the intervention has been successful and reduced deaths or disability. We need to know whether it is likely that these results have occurred by **chance**, whether the results could be **bias**ed by the design of the study or by the inclusion or exclusion of some patients, and also to consider whether another factor (termed a **'confounding variable'**), independent of the intervention, is producing an erroneous conclusion.

Chance and bias are straightforward issues. An example of a confounding variable (Figure 5.1) is the study which shows an association of coffee drinking with an increased rate of carcinoma of the bronchus. In fact it is smoking that is the intervention responsible for the lung cancer and coffee drinkers were more likely to be smokers. The solution to avoid this confounding variable would be to have two groups of coffee drinkers – smokers and non-smokers. The rates of lung cancer could then be determined in both groups.

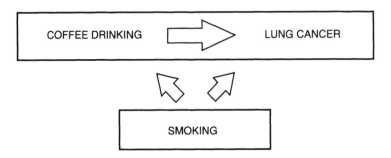

Figure 5.1 Confounding variable

A confounding variable may, therefore, be considered as a particular type of bias, and several biases may occur (and, therefore, need to be taken account of) in a single study. If we were to run a study to determine whether regular exercise lowers the risk of coronary heart disease we might do so by offering aerobic classes to employees of a large company and then measuring the number of coronary events in the groups who did and did not volunteer for the classes. The events would be determined by regular check-ups including a careful history, an electrocardiogram and a review of GP and hospital records.

The results of this (hypothetical) study showed that the exercise group had fewer cardiac events. However, the review of records also showed that the exercise group smoked less. Selection bias could also operate if the exercise group were at lower risk before the programme began – did they have less hypertension, lower blood cholesterol and more favourable family histories? Measurement bias may have occurred because those participants who knew they had had coronary events could be more likely to attend for their study check-up and report their problem. Finally the lower cigarette consumption in the exercise group would be a confounding bias.

Types of study

It is helpful to separate out studies that are observational (and are therefore hypothesis-forming) from those that are analytical (and therefore hypothesis-testing).

Observational – hypothesis-forming

Case reports and case studies

Many important advances in medical knowledge begin with simple descriptions of a small series of cases presenting clinically to astute doctors, e.g. five cases of male homosexuals in San Francisco with *Pneumocystis carinii* as the cause of their pneumonia, subsequently shown to have HIV infection and AIDS. There is usually no attempt to determine causal association in the study – the purpose of the report is to raise awareness. Proof will only be provided by more extensive investigation.

Cross-sectional studies

Also termed prevalence studies (see below), this method involves a survey of a given population and attempts to correlate between personal factors and disease states. It cannot measure cause and effect, nor can it determine changes between exposure and disease. Again, it may lend weight to a more rigorous investigation being required.

Correlational studies

Sometimes termed ecological or geographic studies, these look at the number of cases in a given population at any given time (the prevalence) or the number of new cases occurring in a given time (the incidence), and compare the prevalence or incidence with another population. Limited information as to causation can be obtained but useful inferences can sometimes be forthcoming, e.g. migrant studies of Japanese from their home country to the United States and their rate in successive generations of acquiring the pattern of ischaemic heart disease of Americans.

Analytical – hypothesis testing

In order to determine whether a possible factor really is involved in a disease, or a particular intervention really does improve the treatment of that disease, we need a different type of analysis.

Case–control studies

Case–control studies take a sample of patients with the disease – the cases – and match these cases with a sample of the population who do not have the disease – the controls (Figure 5.2). The controls need to be as similar as

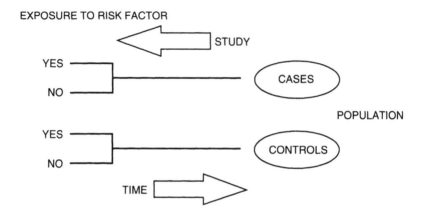

Figure 5.2 Exposure to risk factor

possible to the cases (except in respect of the risk exposure) to reduce bias. The case–control study then looks *backwards* in time and tries to determine the frequency of exposure to the identified risk factor in both cases and controls. The results are usually presented in a table:

	Disease	
	Cases	Controls
Exposed	a	b
Not exposed	c	d

The odds ratio of the exposure resulting in the disease can then be calculated from:

$$\frac{ad}{bc}$$

An odds ratio of 1 would show no association, a value below this a protective effect of exposure, and numbers in excess of 1 a possible association, though a causal relationship would require further consideration in almost all circumstances. It should be noted that an odds ratio from a case–control study is not a measure of the risk in the general population – as an inherent part of their design case–control studies cannot provide incidence data.

Hypothetical results from a case–control study designed to see whether lung cancer is linked to smoking might produce the following table:

	Disease	
	Cases	Controls
Exposed (smoking)	56	230
Not exposed	7	246

The odds ratio would therefore be:

$$\frac{56 \times 246}{230 \times 7} = \frac{13\,776}{1610} = 8.6.$$

This would be a large enough odds ratio to indicate the possibility that there was a true association between exposure and disease.

An example of the usefulness of the case–control design was published in 1994.[6] Several case series had previously shown that in patients with low back pain a magnetic resonance imaging (MRI) scan had demonstrated lumbosacral disc abnormalities in the majority. However, when a control group was also studied a similar incidence of disc abnormalities was found. This resulted in an odds ratio approximating to 1 and therefore doubts being expressed over the hypothesis that the abnormalities seen on MRI scanning in cases of low back pain are related to the cause of the pain.

Cohort studies

In a cohort study a sample of the population who have the potential to develop a disease is assembled (Figure 5.3). This sample is then classified into characteristics (possible risk factors) that might be related to outcome. Observation over time then takes place with collection of data to see which members of the cohort experience the outcome being measured. Cohort studies are sometimes called longitudinal or incidence studies.

Sometimes cohort studies are performed where the sample is selected historically. A good example of this is the UK birth cohorts where all babies born in a single week in 1948, 1958 and 1970 have been followed throughout their lives. The sample is available for follow-up in the present but the cohort is assembled in the past. A concurrent or prospective cohort study assembles the cohort in the present and is then destined to follow the cohort forward, with follow-up at a designated point or points in the future.

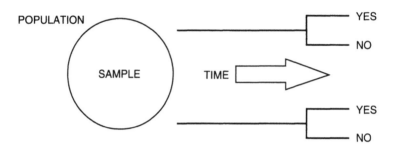

Figure 5.3 Cohort study

Cohort studies also usually present their main results in the form of a table:

	Outcome	
	Yes	No
Exposed	a	b
Not exposed	c	d

The simplest analysis consists of attributable risk (sometimes called absolute risk or risk difference) and relative risk (sometimes called risk ratio).

Attributable risk answers the question 'What is the incidence of disease attributable to exposure?' and is simply a – c.

Relative risk answers the question 'How many times are exposed persons more likely to develop the disease, relative to non-exposed persons?', i.e. the incidence in the exposed divided by the incidence in the non-exposed. This is expressed as:

$$\frac{a}{a+b} \div \frac{c}{c+d}$$

As an example let us consider the development of deep vein thromboses (DVT) in oral contraceptive users. Hypothetical results might produce the following table:

	Outcome	
	Yes	No
Exposed (on oral contraceptive)	41	9996
Not exposed	7	10 009

These results would give an attributable risk of 34 and a relative risk of 6 – significantly large enough numbers to indicate the possibility of a real association between exposure and outcome. However, the possibility of bias very often arises in studies and the risk is greater in designs that are other than randomized trials. In this case, are women at higher risk of DVT given an oral contraceptive? Is it possible that women on oral contraceptives are more likely to themselves report symptoms of a DVT, whereas women not on the treatment will ignore them? Are doctors more likely to make the diagnosis when their own suspicions have been raised by their patient's current medication? These are real possibilities and a well-designed study will provide evidence to restrict or refute influences that may skew the result.

A good example of a cohort is the Framingham study[7] which was started in 1949 when a sample of 5209 men and women aged between 30 and 59 were selected as a representative sample from about 10 000 persons of that age living in Framingham, near Boston, USA. The study was set up to identify factors associated with coronary heart disease and 5127 of the cohort were free of the disease when first examined. As is well known, the risk factors that have been identified as being associated with the development of coronary heart disease are elevated blood pressure, hypercholesterolaemia, cigarette smoking, diabetes mellitus and left ventricular hypertrophy. Since the sample is representative of the population and its size is related to the true population, real incidence figures are available from cohort studies. This is one of their major advantages.

Randomized controlled trials

Randomized controlled trials (RCTs) are often referred to as 'the gold standard' when evidence-based medicine is discussed. This is because their design restricts the biases that may influence the results of case–control and cohort studies. They are undoubtedly the standard of excellence for assessing the effects of treatment.

The design of randomized controlled trials is familiar (Figure 5.4). The patients to be studied are selected by defined criteria from a larger number of patients with the condition under investigation. Those who agree to participate in the study are then randomized (by a system analogous to tossing a coin) into two groups of comparable prognosis. Randomization produces two groups which differ only by chance – the purpose is not to produce equal groups, though in large trials the groups that emerge are balanced. Two comparable interventions are then applied to the groups and the outcomes measured. Ideally, patients, their attending physicians and the

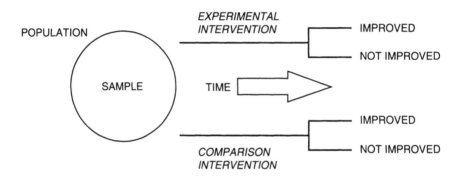

Figure 5.4 Randomized controlled trials

study investigators should all be unaware of which patients received which treatments – a process known as blinding. Both randomization and blinding are used to avoid bias, with errors in the results obtained therefore restricted to chance. Where small improvements in outcomes are expected from the intervention under investigation, large numbers of patients are required for the trial.

Finally, the RCT design needs to consider whether the objective is to find out whether offering treatment helps in normal clinical practice or whether the treatment is efficacious under ideal circumstances. For example, if we were investigating a new antibiotic used for pneumonia we could design an RCT where the outcomes could either be clearance of the causative organism from the sputum or the length of stay in hospital. The first study might show that the organism was cleared faster than with placebo or an alternative antibiotic and (all other aspects being equal) would produce a valid assessment of the drug's efficacy. However, for this result to be generalizable to everyday practice we would want to know that patients recuperated quicker and were able to leave hospital earlier. Conducting a trial with such an outcome would, however, potentially lead to the introduction of other variables (e.g. concurrent or intercurrent illnesses, variations in administration procedures and policies on discharge from hospital) which could bias the result. RCTs therefore often try and strike a balance between validity and generalizability. They may often only answer one or other question, and the subsequent debate fills up the correspondence columns of medical journals.

An additional problem is that RCTs are, by definition, measuring treatment being provided in an experimental (and therefore artificial) setting.

Transferring a valid result from the RCT carries the risk of sub-optimal results due to the different setting and conflicting pressures of everyday clinical care.

Presenting the results of an RCT produces the table below. The results of an RCT are often only presented as a relative risk reduction (RRR), e.g. 'magicillin reduces the length of stay in hospital in patients with pneumonia by 45%'. Whilst the RRR answers the question 'How much better is the active treatment than the comparison intervention?', it does not take into account the incidence of the disease in the population. If we are to assess the value of magicillin to society we need the absolute risk reduction (ARR), which answers the question 'How many fewer patients will get the outcome I am measuring if I use active treatment instead of the comparison intervention?'

	Outcome	
	Yes	No
Comparison intervention	a	b
Experimental intervention	c	d

Absolute risk reduction is therefore the comparison intervention patients with the outcome out of the total of the comparison patients minus the experimental patients with the outcome out of the total patients on experimental treatment, i.e.:

$$\frac{a}{a+b} - \frac{c}{c+d}$$

Relative risk reduction is ARR in a ratio to the outcomes measured in the comparison group, i.e.:

$$\frac{\dfrac{a}{a+b} - \dfrac{c}{c+d}}{\dfrac{a}{a+b}}$$

These complicated formulae become clearer if we consider real data from the recent 4S study[8] shown in the table below:

	Outcome (death)		
	Yes	No	Total
Comparison intervention (placebo)	256	1967	2223
Experimental intervention (simvastatin)	182	2039	2221

The ARR is $(256/2223) - (182/2221) = 0.115 - 0.082 = 0.033$.
The RRR is $0.033/0.115 = 0.29$, or expressed as a percentage, 29%.

Treating patients with established coronary heart disease (CHD) with simvastatin for a mean duration of 5.4 years in the 4S study therefore reduced all-cause mortality by 29%. All in all, a pretty impressive result – even when the particular circumstances of an RCT and the patients excluded from the study are taken into account. However, in order to assess the benefits when the study is applied to the population we need to consider the incidence of deaths from CHD. The ARR takes this into account but the figure of 0.033 is difficult to interpret. The figure contains more useful information than the crude risk reduction but the decimal form is unfamiliar to clinicians. What does 0.033 mean in practice?

This difficulty is solved by dividing the ARR into 1, i.e. by taking its reciprocal. This turns out to be the number of patients we need to treat with the experimental intervention to prevent one outcome. $1/0.033 = 30$. We now know we need to treat 30 patients with CHD for 5.4 years with simvastatin to prevent one death – a much more accessible and meaningful statement than 'the absolute risk reduction is 0.033'.

Numbers needed to treat (NNTs) are now starting to be quoted in trials in the mainstream peer-reviewed medical journals. The clinical effectiveness industry is also busy calculating NNTs for current interventions. Some of these are presented in the table below.[9] (N.B. Refer to the original studies for full details – these data are accurate and very interesting as a crude comparison between interventions, but the full picture from the original papers is required to obtain the nuances of e.g. trial design, withdrawals, exclusions, blinding and other potential biases.)

Intervention	Outcome	NNT
streptokinase + aspirin v. placebo (ISIS 2)	prevent I death at 5 weeks	20
tPA v. streptokinase (GUSTO trial)	save I life with tPA usage	100
simvastatin v. placebo in CHD	prevent I major event in 5 years	15
treating hypertension in the over-60s	prevent I major event in 5 years	18
aspirin v. placebo in healthy adults	prevent MI or death in I year	500

Now the clinical effectiveness picture begins to make a little more sense. We can advocate streptokinase with aspirin in myocardial infarction, treating hypertension in the over-60s and using simvastatin in coronary heart disease, whilst being very cautious at first glance about primary prevention of CHD with aspirin and about the overall benefits of tPA over streptokinase. We need to know more about the particular studies to determine their generalizability and whether there are some special subgroups of patients where the benefits might be greater or less than the population in general, but the NNT allows some useful comparisons between the proportional benefits of different medical treatments and their overall contribution to health care.

Even so, there are caveats to be added. We have not considered the side-effects of our interventions. How many patients with hypertension will develop impotence, gout or diabetes as a result of our treatment? How serious a risk is there of rhabdomyelosis or hepatitis with simvastatin? How great is the risk of causing a haemorrhagic stroke or serious anaphylactic reaction with streptokinase? Further development is therefore likely towards a combined index which will result in accessible compilation of data that will incorporate both the benefits and the risks of interventions, together with an indication of the likely improvement in the quality as well as the quantity of life. Still there will be difficulties in applying these data to individual patients with multiple pathologies and risk factors. But it is easy to envisage, not very far in the future, expert guidance software on the GP's desktop that will calculate the odds of different interventions based on biological data for that patient, patient and clinician then discussing and compiling a management plan based on evidence rather than clinical experience and opinion. Clinicians therefore need to understand how to access and assess information on effective interventions – individual studies, meta-analyses and systematic reviews – and be effective communicators of this new information to their patients.

Two final points before leaving this basic introduction to clinical effectiveness – tests of significance and the advantages and disadvantages of the different types of study design.

Tests of significance

Statistics is, for many clinicians, a concept even more detestable than management. This is due to our own value systems, mathematical ineptitude and the fact that mathematics and statistics are almost always taught by highly competent and qualified mathematicians. Unfortunately, this means that not only do they speak a different language from their students but they also find it a frustrating experience trying to teach what are, to them, very simple concepts. Disillusion quickly sets in upon both parties, confusion and bewilderment are not far behind and another biological scientist thinks understanding statistics is an impossibility.

Having prepared postgraduate students for the examination for membership of the Royal College of General Practitioners for 10 years, two principles stand out when it comes to statistics:

1 Since most of the really important evidence-based medicine is based on randomized clinical trials, only a knowledge of what *probability* and *confidence intervals* are, and what they mean, is required.

2 For those who wish to learn a little more, there is an understandable introduction to statistics written by a psychologist in terms that non-mathematicians can understand. Most medics usually only come to this advanced stage of development after the passage of some time and the internal kindling of a spark of interest by a chance event, rather than being driven by the external forces of needing to pass an examination. *Simple Statistics*[10] is a truly wonderful book and deserves to be regarded as a classic.

Probability

Trials are analysed on the basis that there is no difference between the treatments. This is termed the 'null hypothesis'. The probability that the observed differences could have occurred by chance is tested and the familiar *p* value is obtained. By convention, if a result is obtained which could only have occurred by chance once in 20 times, this is judged to be 'significant'. Once in 20 is the same as five times in 100, and this is expressed as $p = 0.05$. For example, in a randomized controlled trial there are found to be fewer deaths with treatment A than with treatment B. We need to know whether this result could have occurred by chance. Our statistician with the computer software tells us that the p value is 0.001. This means that there is only a 1 in 1000 chance of that result occurring by chance and there is a significant difference between our treatments.

The usefulness of p values is limited on some occasions. A result of 0.049 is, by convention, significant (since it is less than 0.05), whereas one of 0.051 is, by convention, not significant. Clearly, that is nonsense. The second problem is that the magnitude of the differences between treatments is not explained by probability. *No statistical test can definitely prove anything.* All statistics can do is quantify the likelihood that the observed result is a real effect rather than due to chance. Clinical significance should always be considered as well as statistical significance.

Confidence intervals

The confidence interval (CI) around a result observed in a sample of patients in a study indicates the range of values within which it is fairly certain (usually 95% certain) that the result of the same intervention *applied to the true population* would lie. For example, we have seen that the results of the 4S study[8] show that we need to treat 30 patients with established CHD with simvastatin for 5.4 years to save one life. If we apply confidence intervals to the data we get 95% CI of 18–80. In other words, if we use simvastatin in the same way as the 4S researchers did, *in the population as a whole* we will save one life for somewhere between every 18 and every 80 people treated.

Advantages and disadvantages of different types of study

We need to look for studies that produce the strongest evidence in order to provide valid answers to clinical questions. This means reducing the biases which in turn means that a well designed randomized clinical trial will always be the preferred type of study. Enthusiasts of evidence-based medicine will often only consider in their systematic reviews evidence from

RCTs and reject results from other types of study. Experience has shown that many interventions adopted on the basis of evidence other than a well-done RCT have subsequently been shown to be harmful when that RCT is done.[11]

However, the non-experimental case–control and cohort studies clearly do have a place. They are often the only methods that are applicable to determine adverse effects – it would be unethical to conduct an RCT in which the investigators were to expose the active group of participants to something that was likely to do them harm. For example, imagine in the 1950s discovering for the first time that there was evidence from a case series and geographical data that smoking seemed to be associated with lung cancer. Would it be ethical to take 200 medical students and get half of them to smoke 20 cigarettes a day for 30 years and get the other half to be non-smokers? A much more sensible approach would be to construct a cohort or case–control study and reduce the possibility of an erroneous result by limiting the potential for bias. Case–control studies are also particularly useful when an analysis of rare disorders is required.

A clear hierarchy of evidence exists, with RCTs providing the strongest evidence; next come cohort studies and then case–control studies. Figure 5.5 illustrates the influence of bias in studies of the effectiveness of breast screening. It shows that all the studies have a relative risk of less than 1, i.e. screening produces a protective effect – a reduction in mortality in the screened women. The horizontal lines and bars indicate the 95% confidence limits. It will be noticed immediately that the geographical and case–control studies show greater benefits than the randomized trials. Three biases operate to produce this effect:

1 lead time bias – screening advances the date of the diagnosis and hence the survival time, although the date of death is not altered by the earlier detection

2 length time bias – the preferential detection of slow-growing tumours

3 selection bias – tendency for people who volunteer for screening to be atypical of the population from which they come.

Selection bias is removed by randomization whilst the others remain. These details are not in themselves important but they illustrate why caution is required when considering evidence other than from randomized trials.

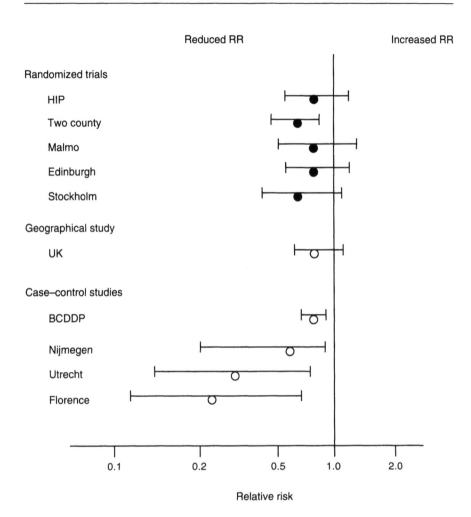

Figure 5.5 Breast cancer mortality in studies of breast cancer screening

Getting appraisal skills into practice

Quite rightly, general practitioners see themselves primarily as providers of primary care. This task occupies most of their working time and energy. They are independent contractors responsible to themselves and to their patients. That professional role and practice loyalty subsumes external accountability.

Exhortations to become experts in everything from child psychiatry to minor (and not so minor) surgery appear in the medical press on a weekly basis. To many practices a 'primary care-led NHS' is the latest trend designed to be the vehicle whereby more work, responsibility and blame will be attempted to be 'dumped' on to them. Keeping up to date, however, is seen unequivocally as a professional activity. The incorporation of new information into clinical strategies, using new therapeutic tools and making appropriate referrals to secondary care for new procedures, is not seen as being anything new. The aim is to practise in line with their colleagues; the challenge is to practise in line with the evidence.

One approach would be for clinicians to become aware of the issues involved in assessing medical literature by a process of osmosis. Numbers needed to treat and confidence intervals are becoming familiar phrases already, even if the precise implications of the terms and their uses seem a little vague to the average medical graduate. Can this be left to chance? Critical appraisal skills programmes and training in consultation skills are now appearing on the timetables of vocational training programmes, and are integral parts of the MRCGP examination. However, their absence from most UK postgraduate timetables is a cause for concern.

Using clinical effectiveness skills in everyday practice can be seen as solving problems and reducing work rather than creating additional strains.

Barriers

- Access to information. If it means a trip to the local postgraduate centre rather than being able to look it up at home or at the practice, how many clinicians will have the motivation and time?

- Environmental factors. If clinicians are spending time fire-fighting then clinical effectiveness will not be reached on the list of 'things to do today'.

- Professional inertia. Is there a will to change the focus of care from responses to individuals based on perceived usefulness to evidence-based practice with individual and population components?

- Perceived usefulness. Are these new attitudes, skills and knowledge acquired of value to clinicians and patients?

Sources of information

Half an hour a week from each of four partners working on priority areas of knowledge for the practice is much more a real possibility than two hours from a single individual. Modem links via personal computers to central databases are the only acceptable solution in the long term. Sources of information need to be credible, digestible, accessible, accurate and up to date. As seen in Chapter 3, many aspects of medical care have been or are being reviewed from the point of view of effectiveness. The Centre for Reviews and Dissemination, the international Cochrane Collaboration and the national R&D strategy are now beginning to produce just such information with the credentials required. Clearly, some work is still required on some topic areas, and there is a need to develop plans to improve electronic access to databases,[14] but if one looks for information of an evidence base on which to treat patients in, say, cardiovascular medicine, asthma, diabetes, maternity care and gastroenterology, then for the most part it is already available.

Therapeutics now has a long tradition of randomized controlled trials. The British National Formulary, drug and therapeutic bulletins and MeReC bulletins all provide ready access to reviews which in any particular area are both succinct and robust. The accumulation of data from a variety of sources has an accumulative effect producing change in behaviour.[15] Supplemented by convincing facts on prescribing by GPs from the Prescription Pricing Authority and clinical pharmacology input from health authority medical and pharmaceutical advisers, significant progress has been achieved in primary care prescribing since they were appointed in 1990.

Uses of Medline

We were recently faced with three separate enquiries in the same week.

1 A practice nurse was setting out to audit a practice's patients who were taking lithium. She was happy that checking the serum levels of a drug with a narrow therapeutic window had to be a part of appropriate care and an audit standard. However, checking thyroid function tests (TFTs) of patients on lithium was the question. The lithium audit pack from the National Audit Centre stated that checking TFTs was custom and practice but appeared to be based more on consensus than evidence. On the other hand, a local psychiatrist had just issued to his patients a cooperation card on which there was a clear requirement for regular TFT checks. Were TFTs necessary or not?

2 A community health council had received an enquiry from a patient with chronic fatigue syndrome (CFS). The patient was concerned that

electroacupuncture for her condition was not available locally and wanted to know why her GP was reluctant to send her for what he had allegedly told her was 'unproven treatment'. Was there any evidence that electroacupuncture was of benefit in CFS?

3 Reversal of sterilization was about to become a procedure purchasable by individual fundholders. They were anxious to find out whether the procedure was worthwhile and, if so, which groups of patients would be most likely to benefit. In addition, was there any information that would allow them to predict which patients were at greatest risk of requesting a reversal of their previous request for sterilization?

Medline is an electronic medical reference database available free to all members of the British Medical Association (BMA). It comes in CD-ROM format which is at hand in many postgraduate centre libraries but is also more usefully accessible to any user with a personal computer and a modem. The BMA library which operates the service recommends PC Anywhere software, but we use the Terminal facility that comes with Windows 3.1 and find this perfectly satisfactory.

A Medline search for the textwords 'lithium' and 'hypothyroidism' produces two separate lists. If these lists are combined a third list is produced of articles containing both terms. Browsing the abstracts of the list of articles from that list showed us that the development of symptomatic hypothyroidism in patients taking lithium occurs less commonly than borderline low thyroid function tests. However, the reports of infrequent but serious iatrogenic illness induced by lithium clearly lent support to the traditional recommendation of TFT monitoring for lithium patients.

Linking 'electroacupuncture', 'VEGA' (an alternative term for electroacupuncture), 'chronic fatigue syndrome', 'myalgic encephalomyelitis' and other synonyms produced no evidence that electroacupuncture had been evaluated in CFS. However, an indication of the therapies that had been shown to be of benefit was produced by the search. We could therefore advise the enquirer of these alternatives and request that if further information that was not available to us at that time came to light concerning electroacupuncture and CFS, we could compare success rates (and study design) with this database.

'Reversal of sterilisation', 'reversal of sterilization' and other combinations of terms produced more than 70 references. From the abstracts it appeared that vasovasostomies could achieve a 70–80% pregnancy rate in experienced centres. An operating microscope and patients less than 10 years post-sterilization seemed to be positive influences. Reversal of female sterilization could achieve a 60–70% success rate. Not surprisingly this was age-dependent, with the pregnancy rate declining sharply after the age of 35. A fallopian tube length of more than 4 cm and again the use of an operating microscope seemed to be positive factors. However, only one randomized controlled trial was found which compared the use of an operating microscope with loupe spectacles, in which there was no difference in outcome (only 72 patients). In fact, most reported case series were of small numbers of patients and in view of the potential for bias it was felt that only a tentative report could be produced, with a recommendation for a systematic review to be performed as part of the national R&D programme.

These three topics took us 70 minutes for the initial location of abstracts. This included dictating letters with the provisional results of the first two topics. The cost of the (off-peak) telephone call to access the database was £1.38. The time can readily be obtained by organized surveying of the medical literature to keep up to date rather than randomly glancing at an available journal when time allows.[2]

Searching Medline can be intellectually satisfying and is a very useful skill to supplement clinical expertise.[2] Like most human activities, the more frequently one performs it, the better one gets at doing it. Inexperienced searchers will miss a significant percentage of relevant articles and courses are available from the BMA to increase the effectiveness of Medline users. Making reviews and electronic databases – including the reviews already available from the Centre for Reviews and Dissemination and the Cochrane Centre – readily available in every surgery, remains a challenge.

The Internet

To some, the global electronic communications system is already an invaluable contributor to evidence-based medicine and consumer empowerment in health care choices.[16] With widespread access to up-to-date information written in simple language, it enables patients to discuss intelligently their options for treatment and select, perhaps with a little professional assistance, their own personal management plan. General practitioners tell us with delight of obtaining over the Internet in five minutes a patient information leaflet from Australia for someone newly diagnosed with dystrophia myotonica, or obtaining from the Library of Congress in the USA a review of therapy for small-cell lung cancer for a patient keen to not only increase her survival odds but to participate in treatment decisions.

To others, the Internet represents more of a challenge.[17] On other occasions, GPs have been faced with requests for clearly inappropriate treatments based upon opinion from virtual user group pages on the World Wide Web. When these include e-mail groups discussing clinical aspects of individual child and adolescent psychiatric cases, understandable concerns are raised.

Whilst increased access to information on health and disease is to be welcomed, interpreting the information and selecting what is of high quality and relevant is as much a requirement of electronic information as of paper-based material. As has been demonstrated in this chapter, whilst critical appraisal skills are not intellectually beyond the average medical graduate, only a minority of the population are likely to be able to find the time to acquire a sufficient grounding so as to be able to assess the evidence they obtain about their condition. Even then, is it possible to be detached about one's own, a close friend's or a member of one's own family's medical condition to make a sound judgement about management? Does everyone want that responsibility? Undoubtedly, some patients value closer involvement in their treatment, but an acknowledgement that treatment is sometimes unsuccessful and the responsibilities that situation imposes on those who have devised the treatment plan, must be an integral part of the plan's development.

If we add on the risks of bogus Internet sites and the inappropriateness of international information due to differences in health care systems, jurisdictions, local clinical expertise and licensing of pharmaceuticals, we can see that the implications of the Internet extend far beyond the technology. As we examine these implications and their impact on medical practice there can be no doubt that the Internet represents a useful vehicle for disseminating credible reviews. More extensive information than is available in the postgraduate centre library is already available with a personal computer and a telephone line. A guide to the quality of information on the Internet is needed, however, to maximize gains and minimize the risks of its use.

Guidelines, protocols and electronic reminders

Clinical guidelines are produced at a prodigious rate in both primary and secondary care. Recently, a general practitioner showed us those she had been sent in the previous 10 months. It was a pile of non-uniform litter, 7 cm high and weighing 1.7 kg. The influence on clinical practice had been close to zero, an experience that has been reported previously.[18] 'External' guidelines, produced without the involvement of clinicians for whom they are intended, without an accompanying educational and implementation programme via patient-specific reminders during consultations, are simply a waste of time.[19,20] In addition, it is now recognized that guidelines must be developed from research evidence rather than from consensus. The latter may simply contribute to the dissemination of prejudice, ignorance and bias – however well intentioned are the contributors.

Attitudes and behaviour towards clinical guidelines in general practice remain remarkably positive.[21] This is a testament to the resilience of general practitioners in the face of an onslaught of material, almost all of which has been of dubious content and value. When the rules of engagement are followed the results can be demonstrated to improve performance. In a randomized controlled trial of guideline development and implementation in Hackney, East London,[22] 27 non-training practices (only seven of which had disease registers before the start of the study) recorded significant increases in the recording of biological data relevant to good diabetic practice, and in the recording of review of inhaler technique and the quality of prescribing in asthma. Electronic reminders also work. Personal experience over 12 years in general practice convinces us, but our case series could be biased! Fortunately, it is supported by a systematic review[23] which shows that each of 21 studies showed an improvement in clinical performance of between 8 and 50% when a computer was used in the consultation. Not surprisingly, better results were produced by targeting onto single preventative measures.

Managing the environment

Overcoming the barrier created by the workload implications of reactive clinical care delivered to individual patients is crucial to implementation of evidence-based care. If we return to Chapter 3 and the hierarchy of needs, we can see that it may be possible by judicious use of management skills to delegate some administrative and clinical tasks currently carried out by health care personnel. The difference between being swamped and having thinking time is about half an hour a day. The environment must be right to enable cognitive and self-actualization activities to take place.

Overcoming professional inertia and perceived usefulness

The introduction of a critical reading question paper in 1992 and a criterion-referenced assessment of consulting skills component in 1996 into the MRCGP examination may well be seen as being key components of progress towards clinical effectiveness in and through primary care. The balance between external drivers of change and motivation for change coming from within the profession is a delicate one. Re-accreditation is undoubtedly arriving for general practice as another bastion of professional self-regulation falls.

Personal experience leads one to be optimistic. When we have been involved with small groups of GPs discussing evidence-based practice there is a sense of enthusiasm tinged with healthy scepticism. None of the skills required are intellectually beyond medical graduates. The flexibility of many members of primary health care teams in delivering patterns of care in the 1990s which are very different from those provided in the 1980s, 1970s and 1960s, leads one to the belief that a further adaptation is not beyond the bounds of reason. The key elements are in place but require orchestration.

Bringing it all together

The steps involved in delivering the evidence are summarized in Figure 5.6. In the near future, as the clinical effectiveness agenda becomes more overt, the locus of patient care remains the consultation. However, this unique interaction has a different agenda. The patient comes with information and requires the health care professional (not necessarily a doctor) to address the ideas and concerns that the patient brings. The expectations of both parties will need to be made explicit and both sets will be addressed, this being facilitated by excellent electronic records. Members of the patient's support group and key members of the professional group may both need to attend workshops to improve their critical appraisal skills and to review guidelines, and they will all become increasingly aware of the importance of communication skills. Many pieces of this new way of working are already identified and available. If the process is clear, what are the priorities?

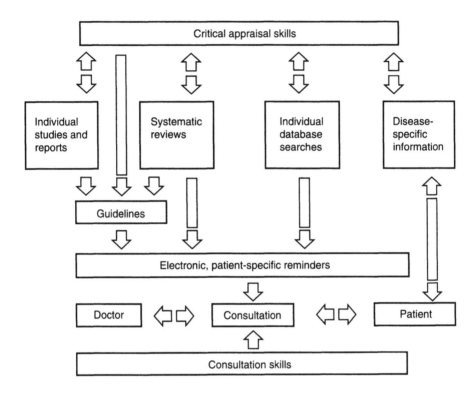

Figure 5.6 'Adding value' to the consultation

References

1 Cochrane A (1972) *Effectiveness and Efficiency: Random Reflections on Health Services*. Nuffield Provincial Hospitals Trust, London.
2 Sackett D L, Haynes R B, Guyatt G H *et al.* (1991) *Clinical Epidemiology. A Basic Science for Clinical Medicine* (2nd edn). Little, Brown, Boston, Mass.
3 Chalmers I, Enkin M and Keirse M J N C (eds) (1989) *Effective Care In Pregnancy and Childbirth* (vols 1 & 2). Oxford University Press, Oxford.
4 Smith R (1994) Towards a knowledge-based health service. *BMJ.* **309**: 217–18.
5 General Medical Council (1993) *Tomorrow's Doctors*. GMC.
6 Jensen M C *et al.* (1994) Magnetic resonance imaging of the lumbar spine in people without back pain. *New England Journal of Medicine.* **331**:69–73.
7 Dawber T R (1980) *The Framingham Study. The Epidemiology of Atherosclerotic Disease*. Harvard University Press, Cambridge, Massachusetts.

8 Pedersen T R *et al.* (1994) Randomised trial of cholesterol lowering in 4444 patients with coronary heart disease: the Scandinavian Simvastatin Survival Study (4S). *Lancet.* **344**:1383–9.

9 *Bandolier* (1994) No.17. Oxford.

10 Clegg F (1982) *Simple Statistics.* Cambridge University Press, Cambridge.

11 The Cardiac Arrythmia Suppression Trial (CAST) Investigators (1989) Special Report. Preliminary Report: Effect of ecainide and flecainide on mortality in a randomized trial of arrythmia suppression after myocardial infarction. *New England Journal of Medicine.* **321**:406.

12 Breast Screening Advisory Committee (1991*) Breast Cancer Screening: Evidence and Experience since the Forrest Report.* National Health Service Breast Screening Programme.

13 Day N E (1991) Screening for breast cancer. *British Medical Bulletin.* **47**: 400–15.

14 Watt I. Personal Communication. Centre for Reviews and Dissemination, University of York.

15 Armstrong D *et al.* (1996) A study of general practitioners' reasons for changing prescribing behaviour. *BMJ.* **312**:949–52.

16 Bishop M (1995) *Medical Interface.* October 5: 1–2.

17 Coiera E (1996) The Internet's challenge to health care provision. *BMJ.* **312**:3–4.

18 North Of England Study of Standards and Performance in General Practice (1992) Medical audit in general practice: effect on doctor's clinical behaviour and the health of patients with common childhood conditions. *BMJ.* **304**:1480–8.

19 University of Leeds (1994) Implementing clinical practice guidelines: can guidelines be used to improve clinical practice? *Effective Health Care.* **1**(8):1–12.

20 Royal College of General Practitioners (1995) The development and implementation of clinical guidelines. Report from General Practice No. 26. RCGP, London.

21 Siriwardena A N (1995) Clinical guidelines in primary care: a survey of general practitioners' attitudes and behaviour. *British Journal of General Practice.* **45**:643–7.

22 Feder G *et al.* (1995) Do clinical guidelines introduced with practice-based education improve care of asthmatic and diabetic patients? A randomized controlled trial in general practices in East London. *BMJ.* **311**:1473–8.

23 Sullivan F and Mitchell E (1995) Has general practitioner computing made a difference to patient care? A systematic review of published papers. *BMJ.* **311**:848–52.

6

Choosing priorities and targeting action

Self-preservation dictates that with a clinical workload of 30–40 face-to-face consultations each working day for general practitioners, a primary care team will need to prioritize the areas of its work which it particularly wishes to ensure are delivered in a clinically effective way. It has been calculated that a specialist needs to read 19 medical articles 365 days a year[1] to keep up with his or her field (and that, at present, the time devoted by UK consultants is under an hour a week). The overwhelming volume of the medical literature relevant to the generalist results in inertia without some agreement to limit the scope of work and maximize returns for invested time and effort.

Strategy is defined in dictionaries in military terms – 'a plan for doing something important, especially in war' – and successful military campaigns revolve around a limited number of specific objectives. The objective may be to take two or three particularly important hills which will advance the cause by an extent greater than simply the territory gained. It is helpful to extend this principle to clinical effectiveness but to do so we need to answer the inevitable question 'How do we select the hills?' Twenty-five thousand clinical decisions a year for a general practitioner[2] are an awful lot of hills.

Linking to need

Providers, in primary care or secondary care, are usually reactive to the needs and wants of the individual. Continuing in this traditional role is not tenable and it is inevitable that needs assessment, linked with evidence of best practice, will become an increasingly important part of delivering health care.

If health care professionals react solely to presenting problems in the way they think works best this may lead to key resources being utilized on areas of health care with little prospect of a return in terms of improved life expectancy or quality of life. This inductive reasoning, based almost entirely on clinical experience and logic with little or no evidence, is no longer acceptable.

In order to compassionately manage the dilemma of limited health care resources and increasing demands from the advance of technology and an ageing population, active measures will be needed. Intelligent service delivery will need to have incorporated an assessment of the potential and capacity of the local population's ability to accrue benefit from a range of interventions. The views of the population themselves on the priorities for service development, perhaps at the extent of withdrawal or reduction of other services of limited value, should be an absolute requirement prior to a change in delivery of clinical services. Agreed management of demand implies an attractive collaborative approach; rationing implies conflict.

Was it really the case that before the NHS reforms development in services for patients mainly occurred at the whim of tyrannical medical consultants demanding new equipment and more staff? And is it now the case that tyranny is now the model adopted by GP fundholders as they exert their whims on the oppressed providers of secondary care? Both accusations are caricatures. On the one hand they ignore the efforts of dedicated doctors, often pioneering advances in clinical care that are today too often taken for granted. On the other hand the commitment of hard-working general practitioners, who have extended their role as patient advocates in the interests of improving the health of their population and providing more services closer to patients, has to be recognized. How can this energy be harnessed to produce maximum health gains within limited resources?

Local commissioning

If the health service of the future is to be successful, the powerful medical drivers of change of the past (consultants) and the present (general practitioners) will need to collaborate with each other and with health authorities. Health authorities are certainly interested in the care of individual patients but have an existing involvement in effectiveness, accessibility, relevance, equity, acceptability and efficiency.

In local commissioning, primary health care, secondary health care and health authorities will need to assess the needs of their local population, understand the evidence which supports or reflects the proposed treatment or services and then deliver efficiently (particularly in terms of access and quality) services to people who can benefit (Figure 6.1).

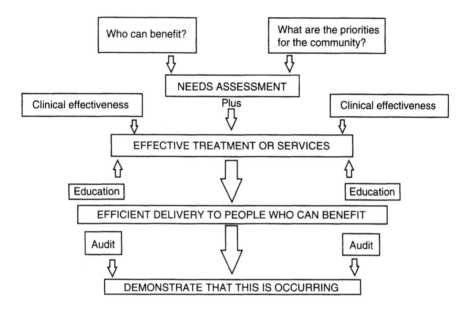

Figure 6.1 Local commissioning

Selecting topics for needs assessment or for clinical effectiveness work in isolation potentially leads to both pieces of work being intellectually satisfying but neither making an impact upon patient care. The art of determining what are the key elements of patient ideas, concerns, expectations and priorities remains in its infancy and will require great skill. Successful initiatives indicating that the various components of such a programme are individually achievable include:

- Dr Scott Murray has successfully demonstrated that an Edinburgh GP can apply needs assessment in a local community[3,4]

- Dr Leone Ridsdale, a London GP, has written a successful book on her personal experience of evidence-based general practice[5]

- Dr Ruaridh Milne has demonstrated that one or two half-day workshops can raise awareness of the place of clinical effectiveness in decision-making.[6]

Alarming evidence of the variations in the integration of patient values into clinical behaviour[7] and in the rates at which clinicians provide interventions to their patients[8,9] are incentive enough for thinking doctors and other health care workers to examine their current practice. These descriptions of major failings in the way that medicine traditionally delivers care lead inevitably to a search for a better way. If local commissioning is to really improve the NHS through GP and patient involvement in priority setting, a synthesis of needs assessment, evidence-based general practice and critical appraisal skills will be required. A change in the organization strategy of health authorities, secondary care providers and primary care providers will also be required to bring these about, which will involve maximizing existing resources (particularly access to valid and relevant data and information), developing the skills of staff and changing the culture from mutual antagonism to collaboration. Health authorities ought to be particularly well placed to take advantage of their population focus, the ability to draw together stakeholders, access to contracting, education, audit, research and development and primary care facilitation.

The Health of the Nation

The publication of the first Health of the Nation documents[10] hardly made a huge impact on either the public or mainstream clinicians. However, the identification of priority areas for improvement in the nation's health and the setting of specific targets (see Box 6.1) for reductions in mortality and morbidity, can be regarded as a key reference document.

The example of heart disease

One of the limitations of the Health of the Nation approach is that whilst the scale of improvements in health are measured with large populations as the denominator (see Table 6.1a and b), the delivery of those improvements occurs at the level of small teams – be these in primary or secondary care.

There may be larger and, as yet, unclear influences that are affecting the fall in the epidemic of deaths from myocardial infarction in many Western countries. Data on 2583 UK patients with ischaemic heart disease (IHD) all under the age of 70 were published in 1996.[11] They were selected as a random sample from 12 specialist cardiac centres and 12 district general hospitals in each of 12 geographic areas. Reducing cigarette consumption, detecting and controlling hypertension, thrombolysis, aspirin, beta blockade, ACE inhibitors, lipid-lowering, post-infarct rehabilitation schemes and

Box 6.1: Health of the Nation Targets[10]

- To reduce death rates for both CHD and stroke in people under 65 by at least 40% by the year 2000

- To reduce the death rate for CHD in people aged 65–74 by at least 30% by the year 2000

- To reduce the death rate for stroke in people aged 65–74 by at least 40% by the year 2000

- To reduce the prevalence of cigarette smoking in men and women aged 16 and over to no more than 20% by the year 2000

- To reduce the average percentage of food energy derived by the population from saturated fatty acids by at least 35% by 2005

- To reduce the average percentage of food energy derived by the population from total fat by at least 12% by 2005

- To reduce the percentage of men and women aged 16–64 who are obese by at least 25% for men and at least 33% for women by 2005

- To reduce mean systolic blood pressure in the adult population by at least 5 mmHg by 2005

- To reduce the proportion of men drinking more than 21 units of alcohol per week from 28% in 1990 to 18% by 2005, and the proportion of women drinking more than 14 units of alcohol per week from 11% in 1990 to 7% in 2005

- To reduce the death rate for breast cancer in the population invited for screening by at least 25% by the year 2000

- To reduce the incidence of invasive cervical cancer by at least 20% by the year 2000

- To halt the year-on-year increase in the incidence of skin cancer by 2005

- To reduce the death rate for lung cancer by at least 30% in men under 75 and 15% in women under 75 by 2010

- To reduce the prevalence of cigarette smoking in men and women aged 16 and over to no more than 20% by the year 2000

Box 6.1: Continued

- In addition to the overall reduction in prevalence, at least a third of women smokers to stop smoking at the start of their pregnancy by the year 2000

- To reduce the consumption of cigarettes by at least 40% by the year 2000

- To reduce smoking prevalence among 11–15 year-olds by at least 33% by 1994

- To improve significantly the health and social functioning of mentally ill people

- To reduce the overall suicide rate by at least 15% by the year 2000

- To reduce the suicide rate of severely mentally ill people by at least 33% by the year 2000

- To reduce the incidence of gonorrhoea among men and women aged 15–64 by at least 20% by 1995

- To reduce the rate of conceptions amongst the under-16s by at least 50% by the year 2000

- To reduce the percentage of injecting drug misusers who report sharing injecting equipment in the previous four weeks by at least 50% by 1997, and by at least a further 50% by the year 2000

- To reduce the death rate for accidents among children aged under 15 by at least 33% by 2005

- To reduce the death rate for accidents among young people aged 15–24 by at least 25% by 2005

- To reduce the death rate for accidents among people aged 65 and over by at least 33% by 2005

---

changes in diets have all been shown to be effective in secondary prevention of IHD.

Given this scientific evidence it is important to survey the extent to which risk factors are being measured and recorded, and the extent of application for the successful evidence-based therapeutic interventions. The index events that patients had to have had to be included in the ASPIRE survey[11] were coronary artery bypass grafting, elective percutaneous transluminal

Table 6.1a: Age-standardized mortality rates for CHD 1985–94 (including target for the year 2000)

Area of residence	1985	1986	1987	1988	1989	1990	1991	1992	1993	1994	Target year 2000
England											
<65 yrs	74.1	72.0	68.9	65.2	61.6	58.3	55.9	53.0	49.6	46.6	
65–74 yrs	1012.3	996.6	972.6	948.6	922.5	898.2	874.9	846.3	808.2	772.1	
Northern & Yorks											
<65 yrs	91.5	89.6	85.8	82.0	76.8	71.8	67.9	64.6	60.6	55.7	
65–74 yrs	1211.8	1190.4	1175.0	1150.8	1127.2	1090.4	1060.2	1024.9	970.0	914.6	
North Yorks DHA											
<65 yrs	71.8	72.6	70.0	64.4	58.7	54.3	51.6	46.6	42.9	41.6	24.4*
65–74 yrs	1080.1	1042.6	1039.7	991.8	975.1	917.8	895.3	842.5	798.0	750.4	642.5**

Source: Department of Health (1996) *Public Health Common Data Set*. National Institute of Epidemiology, University of Surrey.
N.B. Rates have been calculated using a three-year average plotted against the middle year.
* This rate has been calculated as a 55% reduction of the 1990 rate for North Yorkshire DHA (<65 yrs).
** This rate has been calculated as a 30% reduction of the 1990 rate for North Yorkshire DHA (65–74 yrs).

Table 6.1b: Age-standardized mortality rates for stroke 1985–94 (including target for the year 2000)

Area of residence	1985	1986	1987	1988	1989	1990	1991	1992	1993	1994	Target Year 2000
England											
<65 yrs	15.9	15.4	14.5	13.7	12.9	12.5	12.3	11.8	11.2	10.8	
65–74 yrs	321.4	308.0	298.4	285.8	274.8	264.4	255.0	239.1	224.3	212.8	
Yorks RHA											
<65 yrs	18.2	17.1	16.3	15.3	14.6	13.9	13.6	12.6			
65–74 yrs	347.2	330.8	319.5	310.6	298.0	291.4	277.1	260.4			
Northern & Yorks											
<65 yrs	19.1	18.4	17.7	16.3	15.5	14.9	14.5	13.7	12.6	12.3	
65–74 yrs	375.9	359.6	344.8	331.0	314.8	305.1	292.3	280.1	262.9	248.0	
North Yorks DHA											
<65 yrs	16.6	15.8	13.9	13.7	12.0	11.1	10.6	10.3	10.7	10.5	6.7*
65–74 yrs	322.1	303.1	280.0	269.6	277.3	287.1	269.1	239.0	208.3	204.1	172.3**

Source: Department of Health (1996) *Public Health Common Data Set*. National Institute of Epidemiology, University of Surrey.

N.B. Rates have been calculated using a three-year average plotted against the middle year.

* This rate has been calculated as a 40% reduction of the 1990 rate for North Yorkshire DHA (<65 yrs).

** This rate has been calculated as a 40% reduction of the 1990 rate for North Yorkshire DHA (65–74 yrs).

coronary angioplasty, acute myocardial infarction and acute myocardial ischaemia. The results showed that after their event:

- 54% of men and 53% of women had their smoking status recorded

- 61% of men and 58% of women had their weight recorded

- 85% of men and 84% of women had their blood pressure recorded

- 30% of men and women had their serum cholesterol recorded.

At interview, a minimum of six months after the event:

- 18% of men and 20% of women were smokers

- only 27% of men and 29% of women had a normal body mass index

- more than a quarter were hypertensive

- more than half had a serum cholesterol greater than 6 mmol/l

- even for drug therapy the levels of interventions being applied would appear to be sub-optimal (see Table 6.2).

However, the impact of primary, secondary and tertiary interventions must be playing a part in this rapid decline in what remains the major cause of death in the western hemisphere. Still, it is unlikely that individual general practitioners, practice nurses, health visitors, dietitians and cardiologists, when discussing and delivering these effective interventions with and to patients, are thinking 'This will really make a difference to the Health

Table 6.2: Data from Aspire Study[11]

Diagnostic category	Sex	n	Aspirin (%)	Beta blockers (%)	ACE inhibitors (%)	Lipid-lowering drugs (%)
CABG	M	266	91	18	17	18
	F	259	92	25	18	29
PTCA	M	248	94	43	13	18
	F	247	93	50	10	23
AMI	M	249	85	35	28	6
	F	240	86	41	24	10
MI	M	239	78	39	20	9
	F	234	71	37	13	11

of the Nation figures'. Their focus is on providing the optimum care for that particular individual. It is therefore disappointing to discover that the application of these interventions outside of the clinical trial area is poor, though it is to the great credit of British doctors that they were prepared to report their poor performance.

Whilst the Health of the Nation strategy has relevance at the macro level, something more tangible at the micro level is required. Selected targeting of diseases or conditions, realistic approaches and specific audit linked with education are the key principles required to bring about care of patients to a level which is merely in line with known evidence of acceptable care.

Selecting a disease or condition

Parameters to be considered when setting out to develop local priorities are:

- a condition with a high morbidity or mortality. The health gain from delivering a more effective or efficient service will be greater high risk equals big gains, e.g. ischaemic heart disease, cancers, mental illness

- variation from local or national patterns. For example, from Health of the Nation indicators a higher than expected number of teenage pregnancies and terminations of pregnancies may indicate the need to consider a specific local initiative

- major service users. Many major service users are those with high morbidity or mortality. Others (e.g. osteoarthritis) may have a lower profile than perhaps they deserve

- local or national concern over current effectiveness or efficiency, e.g. the *Effective Health Care* bulletin on the treatment of menorrhagia demonstrated the very limited value of a dilation and curettage of a woman's uterus under the age of 40 years.[12] Many purchasers and providers of health care are examining current practice as a result

- potential to change current practice. Tilting at windmills did not prove productive for Don Quixote. There may rightly be concerns about the effectiveness of many current practices (e.g. GP home visiting, cervical cytology programmes) but it is unlikely that currently there will be agreement to a radical change from present patterns of care

- new clinical development. A major change from the present system of clinical developments is needed. Providers developing a service and then expecting the taxpayer (through purchasers) to pay for their enterprise without any assessment of need or evidence of effectiveness is no longer tenable. The need to support developments with needs and effectiveness evidence should increase the pace of justifiable developments rather than stifle them

- be realistic. Even the most enthusiastic individual or organization will only be able to deliver a sensible programme of needs assessment and clinical effectiveness review on a very limited number of topics in any given period of time. Keep it small!

Collecting data

The dangers are:

- being seduced into thinking that because it is possible to collect data then from that process somehow 'the answer' will emerge

- looking at data uncritically.

The following questions should be asked about any set of data:

- are these data about health?

- are they about need (capacity to benefit)?

- are they about outcomes?

- how up to date are they?

- how complete, reliable and accurate are they?

- do they relate to the locality we are interested in?

- how small scale are they?

- will they affect change?

Potential data sources are:

- surveys (disease specific or general measure of health, e.g. S.F.36.)

- rapid participatory appraisal
- census and local authority data, standardized mortality ratios, birth and death statistics
- In-patient and out-patient data from secondary care
- complaints data
- Fourth National Morbidity Survey in General Practice[13]
- prescribing data (PACT)
- health authority data, e.g. compiled from practice annual reports
- GP computer data.

Problems with the GP computer data

It is superficially attractive to look to data held on GP computer systems to make a significant contribution to defining the needs of a local population. Limitations are:

- that data are not collected by all practices
- different practices collect different data in different ways
- different computer systems collect different data in different ways
- data are often inconsistently collected by practices
- it takes time and skill to extract data
- it takes time and skill to process and interpret data
- there are still problems with the ethics and confidentiality of electronic storage
- trust is required between the key players before GPs are prepared to share their data.

Rapid participatory appraisal (RPA) is worth a particular mention. This technique is now well recognized as one legitimate way of determining the needs of a community. In this method about 20 individuals are selected for a semi-structured interview. Volunteers are not requested, rather the interviewers select participants on the basis of who knows about the community (corner

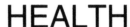

```
LEGISLATION
ENVIRONMENT
INCOME
HOUSING
LIFESTYLE          HEALTH
EMPLOYMENT
GENETIC
CHANCE
HEALTH CARE
```

Figure 6.2 Determinants of health

shopkeeper, postman, publican, community policeman) or who in the community can get things done (councillor, community worker, editor of local newspaper). When the evidence gleaned from the RPA is placed alongside practice data, a postal survey, hospital authority data relating to the locality and census data, a powerful tool for change is created.[3,4]

It is important for primary health care teams to recognize that needs assessment may reveal that other mediators of improvement in health may exist rather than just health *care*. Scott Murray's work[3] revealed the need for better transport arrangements and the local bus company changed the route of the local service. This allowed the population easier access to the local supermarket (amongst other services), leading to an improvement in the available diet at lower cost. Health has many determinants (see Figure 6.2) and health care has limitations when faced with poverty.[14–18]

Making audit work

Whilst the jury may remain out on whether there is evidence that audit on its own is making a difference to clinical practice,[19] it is inconceivable that measuring performance against agreed criteria and standards will not become increasingly a feature of everyday practice. There remains, however, the contradiction of hospital specialists with protected time, training, supervision and greater funds for audit and research, while the majority of clinical care is in the community. Given this barrier to progress, the present healthy interest and activities in audit in general practice is testimony to the work of medical audit advisory groups.

However, concentrating on audit and (for the most part) ignoring critical appraisal skills and needs assessment runs the risk of devaluing audit and mythologizing clinical effectiveness and assessing population needs. All three components need to be dealt with as educational issues, and when looked at in isolation each can be educationally barren.

It [audit] does not by itself provide the necessary conditions for people to learn through it. As it stands the audit cycle is a bureaucratic view of changing professional practice, not an educational one. It is concerned more with the control of people's actions than with helping them.[20]

This may be a somewhat extreme position to take but J B McWhinney in 1989[21] observed that doctors are only likely to change through a process of reflection, personal development and growth of self-knowledge. Audit should be one of the tools for enabling this to happen but is in itself unlikely to effect change if there is a lack of time and/or skills in the other key domains required for change.

Significant financial input as well as blood, sweat, tears and toil has been expended on audit since it became part of mainstream medical practice in 1990. 'Medical' has, by now, mostly been replaced by 'clinical' as the multidisciplinary activity that audit should be is recognized. An industry has been created with journals published, books written, lectures delivered and careers built upon what might be perceived as less than secure foundations.

At its best, audit can legitimately claim to be an effective change agent, improving care for patients and welcomed by intelligent and self-critical health professionals.[22,23] At its worst it can be perceived as an expensive way of taking busy professionals away from their core task of seeing patients, without general evidence of benefit to patients commensurate with the amount of tax-payers' money invested.

The audit–education cycle (see Figures 6.3–6.5), as advocated by McWhinney,[19] produces a process that begins with reflection on practice rather than a set of received standards. Autonomously determined standards emerge which cause the process to be owned by the clinicians involved. There is no reason to believe that this correlates with lower standards. The focus is shifted from information-gathering and systems change towards reflection on the many assumptions which underline general practice. For GPs, rigour is no substitute for relevance.

Collaborative enquiry

The fusion of evidence of effectiveness, needs assessment, reflection on current practice and audit moves us towards new paradigm research or

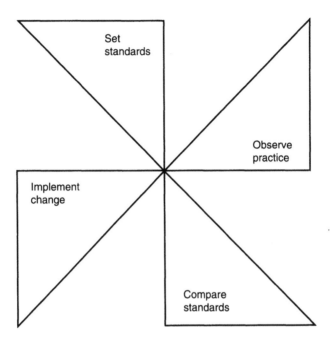

Figure 6.3 The audit cycle

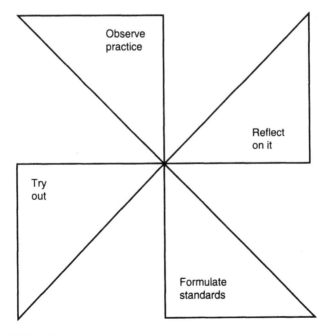

Figure 6.4 The educational cycle

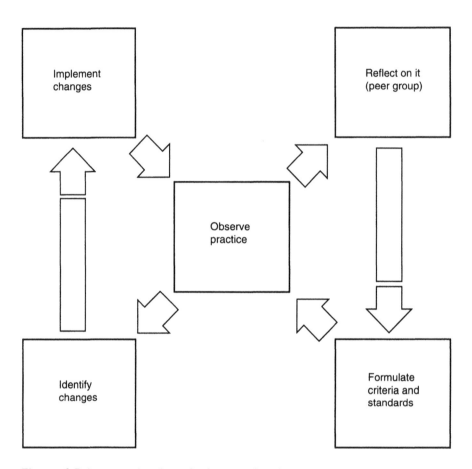

Figure 6.5 Integrated audit and educational cycles

collaborative enquiry.[24] This approach has more to do with the investigation and motivation of dynamic human systems rather than static physical phenomena. Groups of adult learners reflect upon their personal and each other's experiences and problems, whereby outcomes are discovered and tested as they arise. This 'reflection in action' incorporates elements of discovery, outcome results, peer review and learning through group interaction.

Empirical research emphasizes rigour, method and statistical validation of outcome. If these findings are to be implemented effectively into primary care, then collaborative enquiry groups in localities where there are practices collaborating in needs assessment as part of local commissioning of health services in partnership with their local populations, holds much promise.

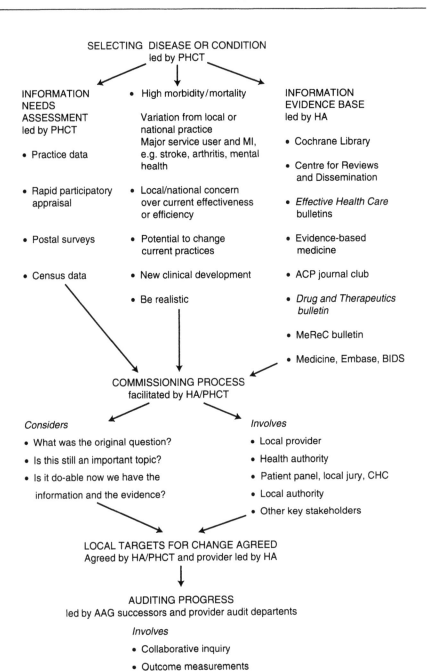

Figure 6.6 Choosing priorities, targeting action

Summary

The process of choosing priorities and targeting action may therefore be summarized as in Figure 6.6. One can rationalize the topics for clinical effectiveness work on the basis of a local group looking for areas of major service use, high potential for health gain or variation from practice elsewhere. A needs assessment process which could be generic or topic-based and collection of evidence to support effective interventions or styles of service delivery would then take place. A commissioning plan would then include all local stakeholders, including representatives of and from the local population. Local targets for change could be agreed, implemented and monitored through audit, collaborative enquiry groups and activity monitoring through contracts. If focus is retained and ambition modest, this may not be an unrealistic scenario.

References

1 Davidoff F *et al.* (1995) Evidence-Based Medicine: a new journal to help doctors identify the information they need. *BMJ.* **310**:1085–6.
2 Dawes M G (1996) On the need for evidence-based general and family practice. *Evidence-Based Medicine.* **1**(3):68–9.
3 Murray S A *et al.* (1994) Listening to local voices: adapting rapid appraisal to assess health and social needs in general practice. *BMJ.* **308**: 698–700.
4 Murray S A and Graham L J C (1995) Practice-based health needs assessment: use of four methods in a small neighbourhood. *BMJ.* **310**:1443–8.
5 Ridsdale L (1995) *Evidence-Based General Practice.* W B Saunders, London.
6 Milne R *et al.* (1995) Piloting short workshops on the critical appraisal of reviews. *Health Trends.* **27**:120–3.
7 Weatherall D J (1994) The inhumanity of medicine. *BMJ.* **309**:1071–2.
8 House of Commons Health Select Committee (1995) *Priority Setting in the NHS: Purchasing.* (First Report, Sections 1994–5). HMSO, London.
9 Audit Commission (1994) *The Right Prescription.* HMSO, London.
10 Department of Health (1992) *The Health of the Nation.* HMSO, London.
11 ASPIRE Steering Group (1996) A British Cardiac Society survey of the potential for the secondary prevention of coronary disease: ASPIRE (Action on Secondary Prevention through Intervention to Reduce Events). Principal Results. *Heart.* **75**:334–42.

12 University of Leeds (1995) The management of menorrhagia. *Effective Health Care.* **1**(9):1–16.
13 RCGP, OPCS and DoH (1995) *Morbidity Statistics from General Practice. Fourth National Study 1991–92.* HMSO, London.
14 Smith G D *et al.* (1990) The Black Report on socioeconomic inequalities in health ten years on. *BMJ.* **301**:373–7.
15 Delamothe T (1992) Poor Britain. *BMJ.* **305**:262–4.
16 Black D (1993) Deprivation and health. *BMJ.* **307**:1630–1.
17 Phillimore P *et al.* (1994) Widening inequality of health in Northern England 1981–91. *BMJ.* **308**:1125–8.
18 Smith G D and Morris J (1994) Increasing inequalities in the health of the nation. *BMJ.* **309**:1453–4.
19 Barton A J *et al.* (1995) Clinical audit: more research is required. *Journal of Epidemiology and Community Health.* **49**:445–7.
20 Coles C (1990) Making audit truly educational. *Postgraduate Medical Journal.* **3**(Suppl.):32–6.
21 McWhinney J B (1989) The need for a transformed clinical method. In M Stewart & D Rater (eds) *Communicating with Medical Patients.* Sage, London.
22 North of England Study of Standards and Performance in General Practice (1992) Medical audit in general practice: I. Effect on doctors' clinical behaviour for common childhood conditions; II. Effect on health of patients with common childhood conditions. *BMJ.* **304**:1480–8.
23 Baker R *et al.* (1995) Audit in general practice: factors influencing participation. *BMJ.* **311**:31–4.
24 Rowan J and Reason P (1981) On making sense. In *Human Inquiry: A Source Book for New Paradigm Research.* John Wiley, Chichester.

7

Realizing the benefits

The foregoing makes assumptions about the intrinsic rectitude of effective health care which few would argue with. However, converting these values to tangible benefits requires an assessment of the redeemable health resulting from their widespread adoption. It is clear that there are benefits for patients and probably for the economics of health care; there may also be benefits for practitioners too, though these may be more obscure.

Benefits for the patients

If the grand strategy for NHS research and development and its practical offspring of clinical effectiveness and evidence-based medicine have any real purpose then the main beneficiaries should be those who receive health care. Uppermost in the hierarchy of gains must be the likelihood that the care patients receive will be of higher quality and that the outcomes of their care will include improved survival and/or quality of life. It is also clear that, in most circumstances, the treatment offered to patients will be standardized and the outcome of treatment will be more predictable and better than is the case now. These benefits are often noted in the control groups in clinical trials. Patients will be less subjected to formal or quasi experimentation and may well be protected to a great extent from unnecessary and ineffective treatments. At a time when most patients, although with increasing exceptions, believe implicitly that their care is the best available, it could prove sensitive to sell these benefits to the public. However, two decades of perceived or real crisis in the UK health service have prepared the public quite effectively for such news.

The growing popularity and use of electronic data, including the widespread circulation of health information and supporting evidence on the Internet, creates the possibility that patients will be better informed than their doctors in an increasing proportion of cases. While much of the 'information' available through this medium is of low scientific value, and some of it is positively dangerous, doctors must nevertheless be able to respond with sound arguments for clinical actions which differ from those promoted on electronic media.

Benefits for the doctors

The greater certainty and predictability which standardized, high quality care brings to clinical situations permits greater clarity of prognosis to be offered to patients, at least in statistical terms. It is often said that patients do not understand the concept of risk; that the odds of survival and its predicted duration merely serve to confuse patients and their families. Nonetheless, they know enough to understand the odds offered on racehorses, etc. and it is more probable that the method of explanation is faulty. The recent attempt by the Government's Chief Medical Officer to define and explain the levels of risk provides a model for professional staff and patients.[1] Since doctors and patients share common interests in seeking improved health outcomes from treatment, it should automatically follow that tangible benefits for patients are powerful intangible benefits for their doctors too. However, there are some advantages of clinically effective care which are specific to, or primarily enjoyed by, doctors. Foremost amongst these is the growing importance of establishing a position which allows resilience in the face of litigation. Even the best therapies sometimes fail and, as the human passion for survival expands towards the search for immortality, practitioners require protection from the irrationality of nature. Adherence to avowed effective regimes of treatment provides a security which litigation can scarcely breach. However, it brings its own risks, for if effective health care is the accepted style, any departures from this path threaten to bring even greater problems of litigation upon errant practitioners. Human fallibility is unlikely to remain an acceptable defence, at least informally, for much longer.

Benefits for the economics of health services

The universal political enthusiasm for the NHS research and development strategy, clinical effectiveness and evidence-based approaches to health care implies an undeclared but widely held belief that the adoption of these principles will help to reduce the costs of government-funded health care. In truth, however, nothing is as certain as this and, while the elimination of ineffective therapies – or at least the restriction of treatments to those for whom they will be effective – may well reduce some aspects of expenditure, others will increase. This is especially so in those aspects of health care in the UK which are characterized by nihilism or delay. A truly comprehensive health service does not have built-in queuing systems (waiting lists) and does not restrict effective therapies for cancer on the grounds of limited capacity for radiotherapy. The impact on health care costs is therefore rather variable, depending on the starting position and the cultural nihilism which pre-exists. A summary of the changes would include the savings from omitting ineffective and unnecessary treatments, the additional costs of comprehensive treatments where these are not currently offered, savings from improved prescribing but offset by bolder treatment in conditions such as depression, and there are the altruistic gains of a healthier population and a better community return on investment from health care. As evidence of clinical effectiveness grows, the debate will switch to the utilitarianism of cost-effectiveness where clinical return on investment replaces patient benefit as the marker of success.

Better clinical outcomes and population benefits

That better and more effective treatment will produce better outcomes for patients is clear enough. What is less clear is how these health gains will manifest themselves in the population. Although the evangelists for clinical effectiveness proclaim massive benefits from following the results of clinical trials, in most cases the benefits are modest. The evidence base suffers from a profound paradox. The major public health issues are common disorders which are treatable (rare disorders and those which are not treatable are either beyond the scope of this book or do not constitute major public health challenges). To amass robust evidence of the effectiveness of treatment for common disorders is simple initially as any benefit is quickly demonstrated because of the large number of cases available. However, all our common disorders are mature and better treatment than established regimes involve small benefits whose importance relies on the large number of people affected. Hence the need for large randomized controlled trials to demonstrate small improvements in the treatment of common and important diseases, trials which are themselves extremely expensive but which constitute the highest quality evidence available on clinical effectiveness. Less common conditions are more difficult to research. Rarer lethal or disabling disorders, for which new and effective treatments are introduced for the first time, are often denied randomized trials for ethical reasons. Only when competitive treatments become available are comparative trials considered and, because of the rarity of such diseases, these are long, complex, expensive and sometimes inconclusive. In some cases, new and expensive drugs such as beta interferon are introduced without clear evidence of their benefits because of the difficulty in commissioning the necessary research, the lack of a comparative effectiveness 'hurdle' in drug licensing arrangements and the pressure from patients for the use of the drug. In short, the best population returns come from small improvements in the treatment of common diseases; the best results for individual patients may come from using new but unproven treatments in previously untreatable clinical situations, hardly compatible with a strategy based on the evidence of clinical effectiveness.

High quality clinical trials are difficult to establish as well as costly to conduct. For the common disorders, outstanding communication systems are necessary, often operating across many provider sites and on a 24-hour basis. Common, chronic diseases require long periods of patient follow-up to establish the full health gain. By the time results are available, the clinical technology has moved on a generation. For the rarer diseases with no previous effective treatment, patients may legitimately refuse to be randomized with the risk of no effective treatment being offered them. Once a new treatment is established in practice, with or without convincing evidence of effectiveness, the entry costs for new drugs are prohibitive and the burden of proof of effectiveness greater than for the first-line drug.

If the community is to benefit from new pharmacological technology, some compromise on evidence of effectiveness is inevitable. Unfortunately, we do not currently have the systems to monitor effectiveness after the event nor to withdraw licences on the basis of ineffectiveness or lack of proof of effectiveness.

Improving prescribing practice

Recent publicity about drug costs and restrictions conceals the reality that the developed world is addicted to drugs of one sort or another. We do not intend to argue the case for legalizing recreational drugs or for criminalizing some therapeutic substances, but the distinctions between them are increasingly semantic. Prescribing rates and costs are rising faster than all other aspects of health care and the measures introduced since 1990, effective though they have been, have served to do no more than to constrain the pace of growth. It is to be hoped that the clinical effectiveness approach focuses on prescribing as the single most common therapeutic intervention as well as one which can do a great deal of good and not inconsiderable harm.

With the increased use of pharmacological substances, the risk of polypharmacy in individuals increases and, with it, the risk of major complications. Most of the 10% of hospital admissions and 4% of deaths which are iatrogenic are directly associated with prescribed drugs. These risks increase logarithmically with polypharmacy as drugs interact with each other and their direct and indirect effects conceal underlying pathology, etc. The risk of such errors is undoubtedly increased by the growing and irreversible trend in self-medication using over-the-counter remedies. However, most such cases occur in people under active clinical supervision.

Conversely, many of the major advances of modern medicine are attributable to therapeutics and this trend is likely to accelerate in the future as new generations of pharmacological research start to affect the market. Not only in the treatment of established disease but also in the prevention of disease progression, therapeutics holds the key to ischaemic heart disease alongside the less-effective behavioural therapies. There is growing evidence that the effective treatment of screen-detected hypertension and, less convincingly, hypercholesterolaemia is having a stunning effect on both the incidence of, and the mortality from, cardiovascular diseases. This, supported by the evidence of the International Studies of Infarct Survival (ISIS) trials[2] showing the impact of aspirin, streptokinase and beta blockers on reducing fatality from myocardial infarction, signals a paradigm shift in the disease profile of developed countries. Both ischaemic heart disease and stroke are diseases in decline in the UK and many other countries.[3] They will be replaced by other chronic diseases as the main causes of death in advanced societies.

As new generations of pharmaceuticals are developed, and the huge profits of recent years are reinvested in research and development, it is likely that therapeutics holds the key to future progress in health care. The need for all practitioners, and especially primary care professionals as the main prescribers, to increase their knowledge, skills and understanding of therapeutics is paramount if the community is to reap the full benefit.

Effective use of health services

Most of the costs of health care, especially those which add value, are initiated in primary care. Most disease episodes are treated wholly in primary care and most effective prevention activities are delivered in this setting too. Chronic disease management, rehabilitation, continuing care and terminal care are usually based in primary care also. However, the elements of care which are the most expensive are those which are carried out in the hospital setting. Reliable data have shown that there are huge variations in the utilization of specialist services by GPs, which are not explained by the underlying pathology in the practice population. These variations, especially in referral to out-patient clinics, admission to hospital as an emergency and use of investigations and therapies, can be as great as fiftyfold in a single area. Without casting any judgement on which end of this spectrum constitutes good practice, it is clear that they cannot all be right.

Examination of these variations holds the key not only to reducing the avoidable costs of health care but also exposing the missed opportunities for effective medical interventions, another example of clinical effectiveness being a two-edged sword in financial terms.

In addition to variations in referral rates, there are differences in the index of suspicion of major pathology, leading to variable delays in referral and, sometimes, to excesses in referral and reporting. It is not unknown, for example, for up to one-third of an area's notifications for communicable disease to come from a single practice or even one practitioner. Most practices adopt sensible regimes for notifying infections requiring public health action. Occasional practitioners notify every symptom which might under any circumstances be associated with a notifiable disease, such as a rash or loose bowel motions. This is wasteful of resources, both the fees for notification and the environmental health resources exhausted following up such spurious notifications.

High levels of variations in referrals to out-patients are not entirely ironed out by consultant assessment. There are also high variances in the propensity of consultants in the surgical specialties to advise surgery for benign conditions. There is no evidence that variations in referrals are compensated for by the likelihood of surgery being performed or investigations being conducted. Therefore, the variations in general practice referrals to out-patients dominate the costs of hospital departments. Most of the variations in costs of hospital services in health authorities are accounted for by the hospitalization rate and this is influenced most by the referring practices of local general practitioners. Thus, the cost of health care in systems like the NHS is essentially the cost of the actions (or inactions) of general practitioners.

The issue of service utilization cannot be confined to health care alone. Increasingly, users of the NHS are also users of other services, including private health care, alternative therapy practitioners and social care services. In the field of mental health, for example, a wide range of non-pharmacological therapies are available, many of them as effective as therapeutics and more so in responsive patients. Examples include the use of substitution therapies such as counselling, exercise therapy (including exercise on prescription) and complementary therapies such as aromatherapy and reflexology. In individual patients these are very effective. The evidence from randomized controlled clinical trials is usually at odds with individual experiences, suggesting that the benefits are dependent on the interaction between the therapy and the patient in non-biological ways. So-called 'n of 1' studies, in which the patient acts as their own control for various interventions, show these therapies off to their best advantage. In the wider context, people with severe mental illness have more basic needs such as housing, income and a social life. The provision of these can relieve the NHS of considerable investment but the complexities of joint commissioning often act as an insuperable barrier to rational practice.

Effective health care, in both the narrow and the wider context, has the effect of reducing variations in practice which are not sustainable in the face of evidence of clinical need. It therefore harmonizes costs as well as practice though, as indicated earlier, the effect on costs is not necessarily downwards.

Effective and appropriate care

Delivering health care which works (clinical effectiveness) needs to be set in a context of the provision of health care which is appropriate. Health care is less costly in systems which are based on comprehensive primary care. Some systems are seeking to reduce costs by introducing primary health care systems. The key moral question in these circumstances is whether the costs of health care fall through the operation of a crude filter between primary and secondary care or whether primary care acts as an efficient filter, allowing through to secondary care only those patients who need and would benefit from it.

On an international basis, it is impossible to arrive at an agreed definition of appropriate health care. Many other developed countries have higher health care utilization rates than in the UK, especially for elective surgery. Furthermore, their definitions of pathological states vary too. For example, in Germany, patients with hypotension (asymptomatic low systolic pressure) are likely to be given treatment to raise their pressures, e.g. salt supplements or vasoconstrictor drugs; in the UK they will not only not be given treatment but will be offered discounts on life-insurance premiums.

In the NHS context, no absolute values exist for appropriateness of care although the *Effective Health Care* bulletins and their siblings are a valiant attempt to help purchasers and practitioners agree evidence-based standards for a growing range of medical and surgical conditions. Unfortunately, as with most of the clinical effectiveness industry, the focus is mainly on secondary care, where the costs are, rather than primary care where the patients are.

The UK has enjoyed comprehensive primary care for several generations. It has low overall health costs, due substantially to the use of primary care as a filter for access to secondary care. However, the huge variations in utilization of secondary care by individual practices suggest that primary care is not a particularly specific, effective or efficient filter and that there are other factors which affect the overall level of health costs. The use of protocols for referral to specialist care may help to standardize its use but it is unlikely to greatly reduce overall average utilization and costs.

Appropriate health care is defined as care which is both necessary and effective; care is effective if that which works is being done and that which does not work is not being done. This is a moving target and one to aspire to rather than to attain.

The trouble with nihilism

As health care becomes more refined, and concern for the quality of life takes centre stage in the later stages of both life and disease, health professionals take seriously the balance of benefit between the side-effects of treatment and the clinical benefits which are likely. This is the legitimate case for therapeutic nihilism. There are still practitioners who do not treat or refer patients with treatable disorders for other reasons, including ignorance, oversight and social reasons. This is so for both routine secondary care procedures, such as adjuvant cancer therapy, and for complex tertiary interventions, such as for end-stage renal disease. There is evidence of institutional sexism and ageism in referral on to higher specialist care, especially in cardiology and oncology; these are other unjustified types of nihilism.

For many years the evidence of these practices has been available through routinely collected hospital data and cancer registries, but little action has been taken. The pressure to raise standards in the examples of these services is overcoming these specific failures but other more subtle discrimination goes undiagnosed, unreported and unchecked.

Even legitimate nihilism is under attack from patients, who expect to be given treatment even where none is appropriate or available. A significant proportion of specialist referrals do not have clinical grounds but are either demanded by patients or made in despair by harassed practitioners with nothing effective to offer. One sympathizes with these situations but every inappropriate referral denies access to specialist care for a more deserving patient. Inappropriate and ineffective clinical behaviour is not justified if it deprives the community of appropriate and effective care.

The Health of the Nation and evidence-based medicine

The Health of the Nation White Paper, published in 1992,[4] set population health targets for ischaemic heart disease and stroke, various cancers, mental health and the avoidance of suicide, accidental death and HIV/sexual health. The general thrust of the White Paper, and the industriousness of civil servants which followed its release, was to emphasize preventive action, particularly through smoking reduction, dietary improvement and cancer screening. Much of the proposed action was not supported by reliable evidence of effectiveness, whereas therapeutic action to achieve similar goals was underplayed.

The most glaring example of failure to utilize existing knowledge of health gain achievable through treatment is in the case of breast cancer where the use of optimal modality combination treatment will deliver the same or better improvement in cohort survival than the most effective screening programmes available. The contribution of therapeutic prevention in ischaemic heart disease and stroke, especially through the ascertainment and management of hypertension, is another instance. The small but still significant benefits of thrombolysis after myocardial infarction and the growing role of cholesterol-lowering drugs in secondary prevention of ischaemic heart disease[5] are further examples of health gain through preventive treatment of risk factors and established disease rather than via the behavioural route to risk reduction.

In the field of mental health, a great deal of attention has been given to the treatment of depression in order to prevent suicide. The basis for this approach is an observation in the 1960s that most suicides had been in contact with their general practitioner in the two weeks before the event. There is evidence of the low diagnosis rate of depression at first consultation, due mainly to time constraints. It followed therefore that improving the ability of GPs and their staff to recognize depression would lead to earlier diagnosis and treatment and a reduction in suicides.

A number of flaws have emerged in this hypothesis during the last few years. First, while several initiatives have succeeded in improving the ability of practitioners to diagnose depression earlier and with greater accuracy, the treatment of depression has not improved. Second, by specialist standards GPs tend to undertreat depression with drugs, leading to patients possessing potentially lethal drugs but still in distressed states. Third, the more recent evidence suggests that (especially younger) suicides are much less likely to be in contact with health services than was previously thought to be the case. Any evidence to support interventions within the medical model which reduce suicide is extremely sparse, skills training for GPs in Sweden apart.

Accidental deaths were included in the White Paper as the focus for building health alliances between various organizations. Deaths from accidents fall into three main groups: road traffic accidents – which are in decline due to better vehicle and road design and reduced speed through weight of traffic; home accidents – including fire deaths which are also declining through safer design of contents; and accidental falls – which are increasing along with the age of the at-risk population.

The most stunning success story in terms of prevention must be the control of the AIDS epidemic. Not only has the number of cases in the UK stopped rising, and at much lower levels than previously expected, but the experience in many other countries is much worse and their decline has been slower and less complete. The evidence on which this control has been achieved was almost entirely circumstantial, there being no opportunity for randomized trials.

The Health of the Nation remains the principal policy on health in the UK; many of its targets will be achieved ahead of time yet more could be achieved if all the evidence available were brought to bear upon the problems identified in the White Paper.

An evidence-based health care market

The language of the NHS internal market suggests that quality and effectiveness vie with price and accessibility for purchasing decisions. However desirable such a state of affairs may be, it is far removed from the reality. The obstacles to evidence-based provider selection are very substantial and include the robustness of the evidence, the (un)reliability of comparative data, the lack of sophistication in the purchasing and contracting process and the strength of the status quo, not least in terms of geography. There are instances of services being moved to take account of the relative clinical outcomes of individual clinicians but these tend to be extreme cases rather than the basis of the system.

One might well be inclined to hope that the importance of outcomes and, more especially perhaps, the application of research evidence into clinical care will become a feature of growing importance in the decision-making about the use of NHS funds and that this will be more readily achieved by primary care purchasers.

The ultimate extension of this analysis will lead to a situation in which the treatment plan for specific conditions is preordained by reliable research, the route to the diagnosis having been similarly mapped. The patient and his or her representative may be offered the opportunity to select different clinicians to manage individual phases of their disease, especially the diagnosis and the treatment phases. Such a situation already exists in many aspects of long-term financial planning such as pensions and annuities; why not in the other most important set of decisions in one's life – choosing a doctor when in need of care?

References

1 Calman K C (1996) Cancer: science and society and the communication of risk. *BMJ*. **313**:799–802.
2 ISIS-2 (Second International Study of Infarct Survival) Collaborative Group (1988) Randomised trial of intravenous streptokinase, oral aspirin, both or neither among cases of suspected acute myocardial infarction. *Lancet*. **2**:349–60.
3 Chief Medical Officer (1995) On the state of the public health for the year 1994. *Annual Report of the Chief Medical Officer*. HMSO, London.
4 Department of Health (1992) *The Health of the Nation*. HMSO, London.
5 Pedersen T R *et al*. (1994) Randomised trial of cholesterol lowering in 4444 patients with coronary heart disease: the Scandinavian Simvastatin Survival Study (4S). *Lancet*. **344**:1383–9.

8

Future prospects for clinical effectiveness in primary care

One of the freedoms of long-term visioning of the future is that no-one really cares if we get it wrong. So much water passes under the bridge that the origins, setting, relevance and purpose of any particular set of predictions cease to be an issue of importance. The worst that can happen is amusement at the error of our ways or, perhaps, post-mortem ridicule. Generally speaking though, prediction, in fields of uncertainty, is fun and low risk for the authors.

The role of the public voice

Publicly espoused values will tend to support and promote the principles of effective health care at all levels, with an underlying reluctance to believe that it was not really like this all the time. Promotion of the genre might take two forms: first, the education of the general practice staff and of the general public; second, the assumption that only specialists can provide effective care, with an accompanying rise in demand for specialist referral which the NHS will not be able to respond to adequately for the next generation.

The promotion of clinical effectiveness in the current environment may be championed by one or more of four constituencies: patients and their representatives, general practitioners and their staff, hospital consultants and their staff, health authorities and other purchasers. The growth of patient information and easier access to the ultimate evidence bases for clinical effectiveness present a new environment in which patient leadership can flourish. There are, indeed, examples of information-led patient influence already in policy-making, particularly in the field of breast cancer management. There is also evidence that patient groups can act with considered responsibility, as has been shown with some of the new but not very effective neurological drug treatments, often out-thinking the professions.

These trends toward patient power can be expected to continue with no real prospect of them being reversed. Leadership by the health professions is rather enigmatic. The leaders of the professional groups tend toward the extremes of the spectrum, the medical Royal Colleges proclaiming themselves in the forefront (because that is where they ought to be) without taking their constituency with them. Local individual or groups of clinicians often seek the other end of the spectrum, seeking to deny the evidence and its relevance to daily practice, or the benefits for patients, or both, and resisting the uniformity of evidence-based medicine. This is true of both primary care staff and of hospital consultants. Each group has its proponents of effective health care and each has its laggards; in hospital the laggards seem to hold the ring. The role of health authorities and other (mainly primary care) purchasers is more complex. It is assumed by many, including legislators, that the purchaser has only to lay down the conditions and they will be followed. Life in the NHS is very different and, while health authorities can promote and resource effective health care, it is only by working closely with the clinicians from whom change is sought that significant progress is going to be made.

A number of potential problems arise from this analysis. Of particular concern is the real possibility of informed patients demanding specialist referral because of a lack of confidence in their less well-informed primary care physicians, their misunderstanding of the information they have acquired or a lack of full explanation of the nature of the interventions required and the competence of primary care to handle them. The abolition of sensible nihilism (restricting inappropriate demand) by primary care practitioners could wreck the economy of the NHS in a very short time as well as compromising the ability of specialist services to respond to (legitimate) demand.

Professional leadership of effective health care is desirable as a less risky and more controllable option than patient-led initiatives. The patient is only interested in one condition occurring in one person; the professional has to cover a range of conditions – a huge range in the primary care setting – but normally has the benefit of experience of several such cases in the past. Here we encounter the tension between evidence-based approaches to treatment (good clinical practice) and evidence-driven approaches (the research-based protocol must be adhered to). Professionals will use experience and judgement to adopt the former approach while the first-time observer will expect the latter to be followed. The best health care is probably represented by a balance of the two approaches. If the professions do not respond positively to the challenge they will have only themselves to blame for the consequences.

The educational challenge

All the stakeholders in the effective health care debate have a lot to learn. It is entirely proper for patients to know more about their disease than their professional advisers, especially in the case of chronic disease. Patients tend to be too trusting and submissive and doctors would have to think more about their treatments if patients were more questioning. For professionals to keep abreast of a reasonable range of diseases presents significant challenges to the way in which medicine is organized and postgraduate training is structured. Continuing education not only becomes mandatory but increasingly onerous for the professional through the course of their life.

The dissemination of massive amounts of information via electronic media opens up the knowledge base to anyone with a modem. A very rapid change has taken place in computer literacy during the last decade and the pace of advance in this area is still accelerating with a doubling of the power of computers every 18 months. Those attracted by the technology are mainly young, middle class teenagers and adults with children, with the elderly being disadvantaged as well as the poor. However, CD-ROM technology is collapsing in price; presentation of this material is improving – one of the key functions of the Centre for Reviews and Dissemination – and it may not be long before the evidence for health care is as accessible (e.g. through libraries) as terrestrial television programmes and Teletext services. Given the availability of the knowledge, our challenge is to help the public to use it wisely; to develop Kitemarks for high quality evidence and research and simple ways of describing relative benefits and disbenefits of treatment options. The days of 'doctor knows best' are over, probably because it should never have been true.

As the day of the patient expert beckons, there will be no hiding place for sub-standard clinical practice. The growing threat of litigation is leading to the development of a generation of doctors who think about the legal implications of any set of actions or inactions; the adoption of evidence-based approaches to treatment is a central plank of such a defensive strategy. It will lead not only to litigation-conscious practice but also to much greater conformity in treatment and consistency of outcome.

The paradoxes of knowledge

As the third millennium approaches, our technology-obsessed population is already starting to rebel against the impersonal basis of electronics. It is frequently observed that the more technology is used, the more the personal touch is valued by consumers. It is essential that these personal interactions reinforce, rather than conflict with, the electronic messages. Those who bemoan the increasing use of technology as heralding the end of personal service by the professions must appreciate that it is change, not redundancy, which confronts them. The health care professional will no longer be the sole source of knowledge and advice for most patients: their role will be to add value to the patient's own sources of information and to help the patient take responsibility for their treatment.

As concern focuses on the style rather than the substance of services, similar changes will occur to life's intrinsic values. As average longevity rises to 80 years and premature death becomes uncommon, far greater attention will be given to quality-of-life issues. Furthermore, as physical ailments impose a reducing burden on people during the more active phase of their life, more action will be demanded on the psychological stresses of modern living. To reflect these changing needs in services will require fundamental changes in the style of service delivery, interventions for stress requiring more time and less therapeutics. The structure of the health professions will have to respond by increasing numbers and changing the skill mix to meet the rising demands of the people for happiness and contentment throughout their longer lives.

We therefore face a future in which paradoxes abound (Box 8.1): effective, evidence-based health care versus personal and individualized care; the ethical safety of withholding ineffective treatments versus the pressure to respond to felt need for treatment even though no benefit is guaranteed or even expected; the risks of unproven and potentially harmful treatment versus the need to experiment if science is to benefit medicine.

Box 8.1: The paradoxes of modern health care

evidence-based practice	vs	personalized care
giving only effective treatment	vs	withholding the only (ineffective) treatment
proven benefit and proven risk	vs	unproven benefit and uncertain risk
nihilism through ignorance	vs	intervention with doubts

The financial aspects of effective health care

There is no doubt that the political enthusiasm for clinical effectiveness has been based on the belief that there was the real possibility that government spending on health services might be reduced or at least constrained as a result. The evidence now points to a rather different outcome, reductions in spending through disinvestment being substantially outweighed by increased demands for interventions which are expensive but which deliver better health. The introduction of new, potentially better and usually more expensive treatments is inevitable in a domain of human endeavour in which investment in research and development (of new products) is rising steeply. These new treatments are going to be used, whether they are effective or not, because the society in which we live thrives on new technologies. We can constrain the speed of introduction of these products and insist that they be subjected to critical appraisal, but we cannot deny that they will, in many cases, be better than those which precede them.

The future appears bleak for comprehensive, tax-funded health care and the need to reduce the financial burden is high on the agenda of all the democracies. They are faced with the choice of restricting comprehensive access, some patients paying for part or all of their care, or limiting the scope of services by some form of rationing. Opinions differ in most countries on the merits or feasibility of rationing health services on any basis which is moral or ethical. The only acceptable path appears to be rationing in a way which excludes ineffective measures.

Defining ineffectiveness is for journalists rather than scientists. Very few health care measures can be undeniably labelled as ineffective: many interventions are ineffective in some patients. Effectiveness is therefore the product of the procedure itself and efficient patient selection, a strategy which requires the full ownership and participation of clinicians to implement.

It has been said that only 20% of clinical interventions are of proven benefit. However, this is misleading as recent surveys have shown.[1,2] The most commonly used procedures are those which are of proven benefit, or at least based on research evidence. As a result, these authors have claimed justifiably that at least 80% of routine practice in both primary and secondary care in the UK is evidence-based. The potential for effective health care providing the economic salvation for state-funded health services in the Western democracies looks pretty flimsy.

The limitations of clinical effectiveness

The large majority of clinical research is concerned with testing individual treatments to treat single disease states. People with multiple, confounding pathologies are usually excluded from clinical trials of single treatments for single diseases. We therefore know practically nothing about clinical effectiveness in people with multiple pathology. As most elderly people receiving regular health care have multiple diagnoses, the prospects for care of proven effectiveness are small although the care they are given, preferably based on research in people with single pathology, should be evidence-based.

Most people with multiple pathology are receiving medication for each diagnosis. The risk of unwanted interactions is high and it is not uncommon for such patients to require admission to hospital with the cessation of all treatment to introduce some common sense into their health care.

As the population continues to age, and health care is increasingly dominated by the needs of the elderly, the complexities of multiple pathology will become the most common presenting picture to clinicians. The purity of most clinical research presents major problems of translation for these situations. It is therefore important that at least the more common combinations of diseases are studied for effective care in real life situations. This may well require a reappraisal of the usefulness of randomized controlled trials for common clinical conditions. What is required are very large inclusive trials, with much looser entrance criteria than are currently the norm, in order to produce realistic outcomes for everyday practice.

The future of primary care

A number of converging themes hold the key to the future structure and role of primary care. Increasing knowledge, of both disease aetiology and treatment technology, will lead the professions and patients towards more specialist care and its delivery by professionals with specific training and designated status. Changing power structures and concern over total health care costs are steering control mechanisms in the direction of primary care with increasing influence over hospital-based specialists. The growing burdens of knowledge, cost controls and infrastructure costs are encouraging the creation of larger practices with the development of specialization and multidisciplinary teams within the practice.

So, the dominant themes are the growth of knowledge leading to specialization, the increasing power and leadership of primary care and the expansion of the practice unit for primary care delivery. The probable (some would argue inevitable) outcome of these themes is the differentiation of primary care. If the situation where all patients are referred to hospital is to be avoided, specialist care will have to be provided in the primary care setting and the training of doctors will have to change to reflect this.

In the first instance, it is likely that the specialists required in general practice will be drafted in from the hospital sector. Quickly, however, general practice will generate its own specialists, steeped in the management of disease in primary care settings but applying the evidence-based treatments for specific diseases of which their hospital colleagues seem so shy. The consultants who transfer their setting to primary care will have to learn about the case mix of general practice and improve case selectivity. GP specialists will have to acquire knowledge, not only of evidence-based specific treatment but also of the limits of their extended competence and when to refer on. The boundary between primary and secondary care, as we now know it, ceases to exist and the role of the hospital service declines substantially. As hospital specialists are used to being full-time employees, the basic ethos of primary care as a self-employed service may change too.

In the longer term, general practice will provide the majority of care which is now delivered in hospitals. Where possible, extended facilities will be available to practices, including multiprofessional support, in-patient beds and investigative tools. The extension of the community hospital network and its integration with general medical services will form the basis of the NHS and will include all community services, some social care, the other primary care professions (dentistry, pharmacy and optometry) and most of what is now performed in hospital out-patients clinics. All general practice should operate in this way and the professions who work in this setting will have been specifically trained in the skills required.

This scenario may take some time to deliver but it provides a setting for high quality and accessible health care which is provided by specialists and is evidence-based. It will be less costly than hospital-based alternatives and will help to ensure that specialist facilities are used for specialist clinical needs.

Clinical effectiveness will be one of the forces for radical change in the way health care is delivered. We must all strive to ensure that it does not become a victim of this nation's passion for structural change.

References

1 Ellis J, Mulligan I, Rowe J *et al.* (1995) Inpatient general medicine is evidence-based. *Lancet.* **346**:407–10.
2 Gill P, Dowell A C, Neal R D *et al.* (1995) Evidence-based general practice: a retrospective study. *BMJ.* **312**:819–21.

Index

Index entries in italic refer to blocks, figures and tables.

absolute risk reduction (ARR) 75–6
accountability
    fundholding 21–3
    primary care 24–5
    specialist services 26
action targeting *see* priority choosing
        and action targeting
Alma Ata declaration 3–5, *4, 9*
analytical studies 69–78
appraisal skills 81–2
appropriate health care 117–18
ARR (absolute risk reduction) 75–6
ASPIRE 96–9, *99*
audit 18, 34, 65, 103–4
    cycle *105–6*

balance of power changes 28
benefit realization
    appropriate health care 117–18
    clinical outcomes 113–14
    doctors 112
    economics of health services 112–13
    effective health care 117–18
    evidence-based health care market
        120–1
    Health of the Nation and evidence-
        based medicine 119–20
    health services, effective use 116–17
    nihilism 118–19
    patients 111–12
    populations 113–14
    prescribing practice improvements
        114–15
bias 67–8
BMA *see* British Medical Association

Board of general practitioners 21
British Medical Association (BMA)
    consultants' role in 28
    general practitioners' role in 27–8

case-control studies 69–71, 80
case reports 69
case studies 69
Centre for Reviews and Dissemination
        13, 83
chance 67–8
change, pace of 51–3
CHD (coronary heart disease)
    age-standardized mortality rates 97
Choice and Opportunity (White Paper)
        23
CI (confidence intervals) 79, 82
clinical audit 18, 34
clinical autonomy 35
clinical effectiveness 34
    equalizing care for needs 14
    NHS Executive proposals 13
    skills use in everyday practice 82
clinical freedom
    attitude changes 13–14
    meaning 13
clinical guidelines 86–7
clinical outcomes 113–14
clinical practice
    unjustified variation in 14
clinical responsibility 29
clinicians
    learning facilitation 36
Cochrane Collaboration 13, 83
cohort studies 71–3, 80

Milton Keynes UK
Ingram Content Group UK Ltd.
UKHW031152141024
449569UK00024B/869